COMPLETE GUIDE
TO INTERMITTENT
FASTING FOR BEGINNERS

By

Zana Aamir

Disclaimer:

The information provided in the book is for general informational purposes only. All information in the book is provided in good faith, however, we make no representation or warranty of any kind, express or implied, regarding the accuracy, adequacy, validity, reliability, availability, or completeness of any information in the book.

Under no circumstances shall we have any liability to you for any loss or damage of any kind as a result of the use of the book or reliance on any information provided in the book. Your use of the book and your reliance on any information in the book is solely at your own risk.

While we have made every attempt to ensure that the information contained in this site has been obtained from reliable sources, the book cannot and does not contain medical advice. The information is provided for general informational and educational purposes only and is not a substitute for professional medical advice. Accordingly, before taking any actions based upon the information in the book, we encourage you to consult with the appropriate professionals. We do not provide any kind of medical advice. Content published in the book is intended to be used and must be used for informational purposes only. It is very important to do your own analysis before making any decision based on your own personal circumstances. You should take independent medical advice from professional or independent research and verify any information that you find in the book and wish to rely upon.

Copyright notice

Table of Contents

Introduction

Intermittent fasting is becoming more and more popular, but it has been around for centuries for many reasons - religious traditions, health benefits, and effective weight loss. With this book, you will be able to learn the basics of intermittent fasting, how it can benefit you and your health and how you can lose up to 30lbs in 30 days. We have included tips, meal plans, common beginner mistakes to avoid, and everything else you need to know, to be able to lose weight and watch your overall health and confidence improve. It is about the change on the inside and the rest will follow - you will be surprised by what you will be able to achieve after reading this book and learning about intermittent fasting. You will learn about the Warrior diet, One Meal A Day method (OMAD), the famous 16:8 method, how to combine Keto and intermittent fasting, and other tips and tricks that will help you change your life from today. Forget the old weight-loss strategies - counting calories and spending hours in the gym and learn about intermittent fasting, which has been proven to give you better results, way faster. In this book, we will teach you how frequency and timing can affect your health and help you make your weight loss goals become a reality.

Understanding intermittent fasting

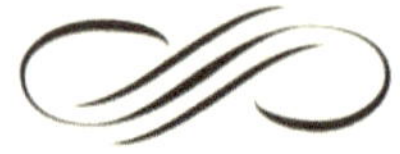

Intermittent fasting has gained tremendous success over the years. You see it on social media, you hear about it on the news, you start noticing that people around you are seemingly losing weight without going to the gym every day, and we can be honest here, you want to know the big secret behind it. So what does intermittent fasting mean? Intermittent fasting involves switching between eating and fasting for a certain period of time. The main rule is to focus on when you eat and not what you eat. There is an hour-by-hour benefit, meaning that with each hour, the more you fast, the more likely you will lose fat, lower your insulin levels and improve your mental clarity.

Historically, humans have been able to go without food for extended periods of time, and often no food was available and they were forced to function without it. Fasting is not just a modern weight-loss trend, in fact, fasting has been around for a long time, since at least the 5th century BCE, when Greek physicians recommended staying away from food and water, to treat certain symptoms of different illnesses. Since the loss of appetite is a common symptom of being ill, it is believed to help us get better, as the body naturally heals and recovers on its own. These Greek physicians believed that staying away from food and liquids is a very important part in order to be able to recover quicker. Later on, during the 19th century, fasting was now studied on animals and humans and during the 20th century, humans were already aware of good nutrition, the type of food they should eat and they had a great idea about intermittent fasting, so they started coming up with different approaches and experimenting with it. Fasting was applied to treat chronic diseases in hospitals and at-home patients were allowed to have plain water or tea that had no calories and that is it - for almost a month and often even longer than that.

For many people, the first association that comes to mind when talking about fasting is religion. Fasting has been practiced by followers of many religions for centuries, including Christianity, Buddhism, Judaism, Islam, Hinduism, Taoism, and Jainism. For them, fasting means reducing their intake of food for a specific purpose and it is still practiced in today's world, during Ramadan, for example. In Jainism, traditionally known as Jain Dharma, (an ancient Indian religion, that is also considered the religion of self-help) people practice different types of meditations and they use fasting to enter a trance state, which allows them to disconnect from the world and helps them to reach a transcendent state.

Most of the Western religions - Islam, Christianity, and Judaism emphasize fasting during certain periods and in India, for example, Hindu sadhus (holy men) are even admired for their frequent fasting for many different reasons. Judaism involves many dietary laws and has several annual fast days, mostly on days of penitence. Christianity has observed a forty-day fast during Lent, which is a period of penitential preparation for Easter, and during Advent, which is a period of penitential preparation before Christmas. These observances have been modified by Roman Catholics since the Second Vatican Council (1962-1965) to allow people to have individual choice, but it is still mandatory to fast on a few occasions. When it comes to Ramadan, Muslims are obligated to fast during the whole month of Ramadan, from dawn to sunset. Muslims eat a pre-feast meal known as Suhur and then stay away from food and liquids.

Only Zoroastrianism - one of the world's oldest continuously practiced religions, has prohibited fasting. Zoroastrians believe that fasting will not strengthen the faithful in their struggle against evil. In the religions of ancient people, fasting was also used to prepare people, especially priests, to approach the deities. Fasting used to be a form of protest and still is, up to this day, used to express political or social views, or can be a gesture of solidarity. There are people and cultures that fast for non-religious or non-medical reasons as well, for example, a town of Geneva in Switzerland calls it "Fast of Geneva", a public holiday in September, where everyone gets a day off and fasts. Nowadays, things have changed and intermittent fasting is widely known as a great power tool for weight loss and improving your overall health, it has been the answer to many health issues and has helped people to lose large amounts of weight, with doctors and researchers declaring intermittent fasting to be the answer to obesity. According to the World Health Organization (WHO), obesity has tripled since 1975 worldwide and most of the world's population live in countries where obesity has killed way more people than malnourishment.

On the other hand, some people fast every day unintentionally and they are completely unaware of it. Let's take a real-life situation as an example. You have a 9-5 job, yet you love your sleep and wake up at the last minute every morning, without even feeling bad about it. It takes you about 30 minutes to get ready and about 30 minutes to get to work, so you should leave your house around 8:30 AM. When you were little, your parents most likely used to tell you that breakfast is the most important meal of the day, but now the time is 7:50 AM and you stubbornly stay in bed until 8:00 AM, because you can. You know breakfast is important, but you also need to get ready and leave the house to make it to work on time. The night before that, you had a nice dinner with your family around

7 PM and you went to sleep rather early. You get to work, open your email and you quickly understand that you have a rough, long day ahead of you and by now, you have forgotten about the fact that you did not even eat your breakfast and it is possible, that you were not even hungry. Have you ever thought about what your body has done while you were sleeping, getting ready in the morning, working until your lunch break, when you finally found the time to eat?

After 4-8 hours of fasting, your blood sugars decrease, you have digested your food fully, and insulin in your body is no longer produced. After 12 hours, your digestive system goes to sleep and your body begins the healing process. Also, your human growth hormone begins to increase - human growth hormone stimulates growth and cell regeneration.

After 14 hours, your body starts to use stored fat as energy and by now, your human growth hormone is drastically increasing. After 24 hours, your body enters autophagy, an important process for cellular and tissue rejuvenation - which drains glycogen stores and ketones are released into your bloodstream. Ketones are chemicals that your body creates when it breaks down fat to use for energy.

After 36 hours (extended fasting) autophagy increases by 300%. If you keep on fasting and go for 48 hours, autophagy keeps increasing, but the most important part is that your whole immune system has completely regenerated. By 72 hours, autophagy maxes out. The word autophagy is not something that we hear about every day and some people have never heard of it at all. Autophagy stands for self-eating and while that may sound bad, it is actually a good thing. When we eat non-stop, autophagy is never allowed to take place. Our bodies contain trillions of different cells and when we have reached autophagy, there are a lot of unwanted cells we are getting rid of, therefore, our bodies are doing a full clean-up, cleaning out toxins and unwanted molecules. If we do not stay away from food for a certain period of time, this never happens. If the only time where we do not consume food is when we go to sleep, autophagy never happens. Does not sound too good at all, does it? Look at it like this. How energized do you actually feel after eating? If you consume three or more meals a day, do you even feel energized at all? Unless you spend many, many hours in the gym, every single day, then trust me, you do not need that much food. We were made to believe that we have to eat for energy, but the reality is different. Food can be the best and the worst medicine at the same time and it all depends on you and how you see it. There is no correct way to do it and this is why intermittent fasting can work and be the answer to many of your questions, because you design your own schedule and eating pattern, it is up to you to choose the time of when to eat and when not to eat. We feel way better when we decide to clean our closet and organize our clothes - give some of the clothes to charity, throw some out, to be able to buy new ones.

Intermittent fasting works the same way - we get rid of the old and the bad stuff and we give our bodies a much-needed detox, to create new cells. It is not advised to fast longer than 72 hours, however, if you decide to do it, a doctor should be consulted.

From a medical standpoint, many health issues are caused by excess fat - this includes diabetes, heart disease, high blood pressure, kidney disease, certain types of cancer, and breathing problems. But there are many people who do not have excess fat, yet they are still metabolically unhealthy, so it is amazing that people would rather choose drastic diets and spend hundreds of dollars on diet experts, but fail to understand that intermittent fasting could solve all of these problems and more, just by giving your body and your digestive system a break and following a simple eating pattern. Studies show that intermittent fasting, when done right, can be an effective tool for major health benefits. Fasting improves your mental clarity - you will notice that it is easier for you to focus, you will feel way more energized and of course, the best part is seeing the obvious weight loss and health improvement right away. There are plenty of studies, books, and researches are done on how to improve your health by eating healthy, exercising, counting calories, and avoiding certain foods, but these things often lead to bad consequences, slowing your metabolism and make you binge-eat, after limiting yourself and trying to avoid certain cravings. You are probably wondering: "Do I really just have to skip breakfast and I will lose fat, without working out?" Truth be told, the answer is yes. Let us make it even more interesting for you. Did you know that you can lose fat by eating bacon? Next to some scrambled eggs, which has spent a decent amount of time in butter on your pan and a big cup of coffee with heavy cream or butter in it? It probably sounds improbable and you may feel like you have been lied to all your life, because how do you lose weight by eating bacon? For instance, in order to lose weight, you probably count calories and eat nothing but spinach and celery all day long, to see the results you have been wanting to see for a long time, but this has not been beneficial. We have been taught that this is how it is supposed to be - we have to eat breakfast, we have to eat at least 3 times a day, add some workouts on top and we will be fine.

It does not always work that way and that does not always mean that you will be able to maintain your current weight or lose weight. There is something that dietitians, doctors, and these diet books have in common and we have all heard about it - do not eat after 6 PM. But no one has really explained why or what that even means for you. No one has mentioned that this is directly related to intermittent fasting, and well… it is. These books will tell you to count calories, eat super healthy, but you should stop eating at a certain time, meaning that the whole world has agreed on one thing - it is important when you eat. But what about the other part, the "how you eat" part. A lot of these books do not mention the fact that you will feel extremely hungry after eating greens and nothing but vegetables all day, you will feel pretty miserable and want to give up on the diet and just go and make the sandwich you have been dreaming about all day long.

Eating throughout the day and not giving your body a break at all, will often make you feel bloated and uncomfortable, but it is possible that you are used to this and you may not even notice it anymore, it has become a norm for you. Let me tell you, your body is struggling. Food coma, the itis, whatever you may call it, is not how it should be. Food is supposed to give you energy and not make you feel sleepy after a meal. So why do we feel like we should take a nap after lunch, or why are we so unproductive at work, after coming back from lunch and we do not feel like working or doing anything at all? And then we look around and see that everyone is drowsy and sleepy and it almost feels like everyone and everything is stuck? Why choose that and not feel energized and in control of your body? Wouldn't it be nice to feel energized and focused during the day, not have any uncomfortable stomach issues, and enjoy your sleep to the fullest, because your body is not trying to deal with the terrible decisions you have made throughout the day? It's not one of those "too good to be true" scenarios. Intermittent fasting can suit your needs, your lifestyle, your habits, and your schedule. The best part is that you are in full control of it. During these fasting periods, you either eat very little or nothing at all, but during your eating window - it is your choice, whether you want to cut down on carbs and choose the Ketogenic diet, or you want to consume less than 1000 calories for two days a week and eat normally for the other 5 days (the 5:2 method) or you want to go all out and have a nice meal once a day, without restricting yourself at all. Remember, the same thing will not work for everyone and that is the beauty of intermittent fasting - you can change it however you want it and adjust it, and still be able to achieve your weight loss goals, by following some very simple intermittent fasting rules.

There is a famous saying that says: "Watch the clock, not the scale" and it could not be any more true. Scales are and will be your worst enemy when it comes to intermittent fasting. It is advisable to do bi-weekly, or even monthly weigh-ins, and it should not be done every day, as some people tend to lose motivation when they see their weight going up because of water weight, or they have high expectations and do not meet them right away. What you should focus on is what you see in the mirror, how your clothes start to fit better, the inches you are losing and the extremely light feeling you will start to experience, as you are burning more and more fat. The reason why intermittent fasting is so effective is very simple. If we look at how long it takes us to digest food, letting our bodies take a break only makes sense. When it comes to liquids, digestion takes about 15-30 minutes, fruits can take up to 40 minutes. Vegetables take up to an hour, grains and beans can take up to even 3 hours and animal proteins, such as eggs, fish, meat, and dairy take up to 5-6 hours. Now let's imagine that breakfast is the most important meal of the day and we decide to have scrambled eggs, bacon, and toast for breakfast. This will take about 5 hours for our bodies to digest, but before we are done with that, we may already be thinking about what we are going to eat for lunch. We decided to go for a creamy chicken Alfredo pasta, which will take the same amount of time to digest, the same way our breakfast did. Our bodies are really struggling by now, but before dinner is ready, we also want to have a snack, while watching a football game, or spending time with our friends and family. Dinner time comes and we are having steak and roasted potatoes and a glass of wine. Guess what? This will also take about 4-5 hours to digest and throughout the day, our digestive system has been constantly working and digesting food, without any breaks. Compare that to a 14-hour shift, with barely having any breaks - feels terrible! Your body requires a high amount of energy and your body deserves a well-deserved break. Enjoy your morning without having to stress about cooking breakfast and being late for work, or simply eat your dinner at 5 PM and enjoy breakfast at 9 AM if you want to, because you have given your body a much-needed break, after a heavy meal such as dinner.

Intermittent fasting has a few rules, but doing the same thing every day is not one of them. It is advised to mix and match, to avoid a weight loss plateau - a period of stalling, or even gaining weight. Your body will adapt, but after a while, you might reach a plateau and you will notice that your weight has been the same and you are not seeing any changes, especially compared to how quickly you were able to see progress before. You will not see any fat loss. Sometimes having cravings and listening to your body can get you out of this stage and be an absolute necessity to continue with intermittent fasting, in order to reach your goals. It is important to listen to your body and avoid hitting a plateau at all costs and if it does happen, all you need to do is to understand the main reason behind it and get out of it. It is very possible to reach a plateau, simply by overeating. For example, doing OMAD (One meal a day, the 23:1 method), rewarding yourself with a huge amount of carbohydrates, unhealthy fats, and little to no protein, may not be the best option, as it is proven that consuming junk food, will most probably make you crave those bad carbs and unhealthy fats way more during your 23 hour fasting period and it will be extremely hard to stay on track. There are many ways to enjoy the food that you love by doing it the right way, without having bad cravings and wanting to give up. Once you realize how many things you can eat and still lose weight, you will quickly understand that you are in full control of your body and your life, you will understand that you can lose weight without having to worry about gaining it back and still enjoy food at the same time. Intermittent fasting should not be seen as a diet, whether you choose to fast for 18 hours, 23 hours, or two days, intermittent fasting becomes a way of life. You train your body and your mind at the same time and these changes lead to amazing things. And the best part of it all, intermittent fasting is completely free.

Forget the supplements, forget the expensive dietitian consultations, forget the weight loss procedures that give you false hope to lose 2 inches off of your waist, after 8 procedures. You can do it yourself and then you can motivate and inspire others.

It is important to remember that weight loss and fat loss are two very different things. All of us have heard about the magical weight loss pills that will help you lose 10lbs in a few days and we fall for it, of course, because it sounds amazing. Right? The truth behind these amazing pills is nothing but water weight that you will lose during these few days and while it will make you really happy once you get on the scales, but you have to keep in mind that this is not fat you have lost. 50-60% of our total body weight is just water and our eating habits can lead to cells absorbing large amounts of water just like a sponge. Water weight and the whoosh effect mean that your fat cells fill up with water and you are seemingly gaining weight, but when the cell releases the water, the cell shrinks and you have lost fat. It is extremely important to keep hydrated, as your body will start storing water if you will be dehydrated and it can make you feel bloated. Water levels can make your weight fluctuate by 2-4lbs in one day, so in all honesty, you should trust the process, and then you will start noticing that you will feel a lot lighter and see the weight coming off of you.

Are you wondering what happens to your body while you are sleeping? Sleep and intermittent fasting go hand in hand. Sleep, in general, is a very important part of our daily lives, and it is also a very important part while fasting and it can be considered as a secret weapon. The same way sleep boosts your immune system, puts you in a better mood, increases your productivity, strengthens your heart, is the same way that intermittent fasting improves your mental and physical health. Not only because fasting will make you sleep better, but you are fasting while you are sleeping, so the more you sleep, the more you fast without even thinking about food. It is possible that your eating window might be around 3-4 AM, depending on your schedule, but eating before going to sleep is definitely not advised. Late-night snacks are considered an extra meal and can lead to serious health issues and it is proven that the calories you have consumed before sleeping, will most likely be stored as fat. Your body is preparing to shut down before you go to sleep, so these cravings should be avoided at all costs. This is when the power of intermittent fasting comes into play again - simply by working around the clock. It is not easy to break out of habits such as opening the refrigerator before going to sleep, to make a quick sandwich. We are not here to tell you that you should not eat before going to sleep, we are here to explain the reason behind weight gain and to teach you how to involve intermittent fasting into your daily routine the right way and you will break out of these habits naturally. You will not be craving that sandwich, because your body will adapt to your new lifestyle and if you eat a nutritious meal or two, or even three during your eating window, you will be more than good to go. The thing is, you might not even be hungry, hunger is a habit - it often arises around the time that you would usually eat. But when you reduce the frequency of when you eat, hunger disappears. Hunger does not equal starvation, in fact, your body can go for 8 to 21 days without any food. Hunger can be a signal from your body or your brain or both, but it does not always mean that you need to run to the kitchen immediately and you are going to die if you do not feed yourself. You can be perfectly fine with drinking some water, or green tea without anything added and you will notice that you will not even feel hungry anymore. Or you can ignore it completely and you will be amazed that after a while, you will not be hungry at all, because you are not starving - your body just gave you a signal to eat and you did not fall for it. Intermittent fasting is all about self-discipline and understanding what your body really needs and wants, live to eat, not eat to live. Do not fear hunger, as it will not increase until it becomes impossible to do your daily activities, hunger actually tends to decrease while you are fasting, because your body switches fuel sources. Glucose is the main energy source after you eat, but if you have not had any food and have been fasting, the main energy source will be the stored fat in your body, because you have entered ketosis and your body uses fat to give you energy. No wonder the Keto diet is called a fat-burning machine, because your body does the work for you, and if you make fasting your lifestyle, you will start noticing that you are not even able to consume as much food anymore and therefore, you will consume fewer calories naturally, without having to count it.

Many people compare intermittent fasting to other diets. The truth is, it cannot even be compared. They can all help you lose weight, but one can impact your health in a bad way, the other can only improve it. One can help you lose weight, but the other can help you to maintain it. There is the rice diet that tells you that you should eat nothing but rice, or rice with plain yogurt for 3 days straight, or an egg diet that promises you to lose weight quickly, but these diets are not sustainable and the weight will come back quickly. Furthermore, if you eat only eggs or rice for days or even weeks, your body will be malnourished and you will feel terrible, as your body is not getting all the needed nutrients. Since intermittent fasting will become a way of life, without even you noticing it, so you will be able to successfully maintain your goal weight and once you have achieved it, you can adjust your eating time once again. But what if self-doubt comes into play? What if you feel like you will miss out on your social life when your friends offer you to go out for dinner and you are only supposed to eat the next day at 2 PM? What if you have to cook for your family, but restrict yourself from eating dinner with them? What if you do not reach the goal? These kinds of doubts are very normal and there is nothing wrong with it. It is okay to feel like it will not work for you, or you will not be able to do it. But think about how many situations you have been in during your life, where you have felt like you cannot do something, and then think about the times when you did it. Think about where you will be in a year if you start taking matters into your own hands and introduce fasting into your life right now.

Think about the health benefits and the number of compliments you will receive, once you start losing weight. Or how your shopping sprees will bring a different kind of joy to you because you are not struggling to find your size anymore and you can wear clothes you felt like you could not wear before. The most exciting part is that you do not need to do much to achieve these goals, but simply understand how intermittent fasting can work with your schedule and lifestyle.

Why intermittent fasting?

It takes a lot of work to monitor what you eat and how much you eat. It is a hassle to count calories, some people even weigh their food, to make sure they do not go over the

allowed amount of food and if we think about it, food has taken over their life in a way. They have to put so much thought into this and it comes with a lot of stress and can lead to giving up and getting demotivated, and that can turn into an emotional eating marathon. We should not let food take over our lives, that is exactly why intermittent fasting has been a life-saver for so many people. Of course, the beginning is always hard, you will feel like you are punishing yourself if you really want to get some take-away after you have promised yourself that you are going to commit to this, but once you get over it and eat during your eating window while including enough fat and protein, you will be extremely proud of yourself and the fact that you are not going to feel hungry after a while, as you learn how to ignore it and overcome it. If you feel like not eating for 16 hours is too much for you, you can change it however you want to change it.

Go for a 12-hour eating window and fast for the next 12 hours, you can then work your way up, or involve Keto and reduce carbs, eat more fatty foods and let your body do the work for you, because once you are in ketosis and you keep your carb intake below at least 50 grams per day (ideally, 20-30 grams per day) your body will turn into a fat-burning machine and you will not feel like you are punishing yourself anymore. Your options with intermittent fasting are limitless and you decide what to do and what not to do, unlike diets that are telling you what to do, what to eat, and focuses on nothing but restricting yourself. This kind of freedom has allowed people to stay healthy, lose fat and still eat the things they want to eat. It sounds like a dream come true, but the only difference between intermittent fasting and unhealthy diets is the fact that fasting will make this dream a reality.

Once you take time to understand your current habits, your lifestyle choices, and the way you eat now, it will be easy to understand how to involve intermittent fasting and by the time you are done reading this book, it will probably be the right time to choose which method will work for you the best. Although you should not focus on one thing and one thing only, you have to start somewhere and you can always come back to this, switch it up and try something else. Many people that have tried fasting for a month, either to see what the hype is about, to monitor what happens during that month, to see how much weight they have lost, or do it simply for a YouTube video - will all tell you one thing. It worked. They have lost a lot of weight, they have noticed many health benefits, they have been sleeping better and feeling better. So how come that people are still making unhealthy decisions, eating and snacking throughout the day, even during the night, and not wanting to make better decisions and healthier choices? Not everyone has self-discipline and not everyone wants to restrict themselves, but it is true that not everyone understands the bigger picture here and that this is a lifestyle, not a self-restricting diet or a quick fix. It should not be something you try out for a month or fast until you have gained your goal weight. Our bodies are designed to recognize the changes we make in our diet, our eating and sleeping patterns. Once you introduce intermittent fasting into your life, you should not confuse your body by doing something different every month, because that can lead to health problems. You have to stay committed and we all know that consistency brings results. You cannot do that with rice or an egg diet, because how do you stay consistent with eating nothing but that? Apart from missing important vitamins, most likely, you will end up at the hospital sooner than you think. When we are not consuming what we need to stay alive, our bodies start prioritizing main functions and switching some functions off. For example, if we do not get the vitamins and nutrients we need, we might be full from what we ate, but we could be feeling cold, or experience fatigue and tiredness. If your main goal is to lose weight no matter what it takes and these quick weight loss diets look very appealing, try to think about what will happen to you on the inside and how you are damaging your health just by trying to lose fat, when in reality, it can be done in a healthy way and without having to say goodbye to your favorite foods.

It is easy to see why intermittent fasting is becoming more and more popular. You can go out to eat and not worry about having to count calories, you can have a bag of chips that you are craving, you can have those three huge slices of pizza and you do not have to make yourself feel bad about how you have failed yourself and the diet you are trying to follow. If you think about it, if you decide to have pizza at 12 PM and then have a cheesy chicken casserole for dinner at 6 PM, have a dessert afterward and fast from 8 PM till 12 PM the next day, you have gone for 16 hours of fasting and during these 16 hours, your body has started to use stored fat for energy and your human growth hormone has increased as well. The next day, you are probably really looking forward to your meal and your portion will be as big as it usually is, but before you are done, you will notice that you are already full and there is some food still left on the plate. You have two choices - you either continue and eat it all, because, well, it is on your plate and it still looks really good, or you stop because you are full and every next bite will be a struggle. If you stop and do the same thing during dinner, you have already consumed way fewer calories than you usually do and especially if you have been doing a good job at drinking water while in a fasting state. This means that you have eaten what you wanted to eat, you were not forced to cook a healthy vegetable soup for yourself and cook something else for your family, you were able to eat fewer calories naturally, without having to count them and you are still losing weight because you focused on when you eat, not how you eat.

Do not listen to what people will tell you, you are not going to starve yourself if you decide to introduce intermittent fasting into your life. You will not lose muscle mass and your metabolism will not slow down, it is quite the opposite - studies have shown that intermittent fasting boosts your metabolism and you will be able to burn fat way faster. There are many myths surrounding intermittent fasting, but often can be very misleading. Intermittent fasting does not promote food deprivation, it is a philosophy that focuses on breaks from food, to let your body rest and reset. There is another great benefit that will come with fasting and that is - staying young. There is scientific evidence that proves that intermittent fasting can keep you in a youthful state. Fasting can activate life-extending mechanisms, benefit your skin, create new cells, reduce inflammation and increase the level of antioxidants and oxidative stress can influence the rate at which we age. In other words, intermittent fasting has so many benefits, it is hard to find a reason why someone would not do it. While it is amazing, it is also true that some people should stay away from fasting, at least for now and that includes people with eating disorders because fasting can trigger it, as well as pregnant women, as it is not advised to abstain from food for longer periods of time and pregnant women should not be losing weight - one of intermittent fasting great benefits.

Life revolves around eating and as sad as it is, it is true. From family gatherings to religious holidays and different kinds of celebrations, what's going to be on the table is usually the main concern. Thanksgiving is all about roast turkey, mashed potatoes, pumpkin pie, and all the other amazingly delicious food. People start preparing the food days before, eat all day on the actual Thanksgiving day and since there is so much food left, the family would gather around the next day and eat again. But as much as we were designed to eat, we were designed to fast as well, we already do it every night, but we have missed the bigger picture and gotten the whole idea wrong. Food gives us comfort, but we were not designed to be that way - food is supposed to be a fuel to give us the energy that powers our brain, heart, and other major parts of our bodies.

Too much food can destroy our bodies and lead to weight gain, strokes, diabetes, you name it. If starving is the first thing that comes to your mind when you hear the word fasting, or you think that is just something that only religious people do, you will learn that fasting can be an answer to many issues you have been dealing with for your whole life and there definitely is a type of fast that will work for you, it does not have to be intimidating. If more people understood that fasting has been around for centuries and is something our ancestors practiced every day and it is highly likely that we have at least one person in our circle that fasts without even knowing it, we can do it as well. There are no quick fixes, there are no magic diets that can help you the way intermittent fasting can. Our bodies have told us to fast, but we did not even know that there is a word for it. When most of us get really sick, most likely, we have little to no appetite at all. It is because our bodies are fighting a virus and the last thing we want is to let our bodies deal with a virus and digest a large meal. It is crucial to listen to our bodies and what it is trying to tell us.

Health benefits

It is known that intermittent fasting can improve your health, unlike any diet can. We have mentioned many health benefits, but let us take a greater look at what actually happens during a fast and what are the main evidence-based long-term benefits. When we eat, the calories from the food are stored in our body in the form of glycogen (an important fuel reserve). When the glycogen reserves are filled, the rest of the calories are stored as fat. In today's world, if we consume three or more meals a day, our glycogen reserves are always full and we never get to the burning fat part. So what happens when we stop eating? Our glycogen reserves have been cleaned out and our bodies have no choice but to take fat to produce energy. If you stick to intermittent fasting, you will lose weight and that is a fact. By the time your metabolism has improved, (and fasting does exactly that) you are losing weight even faster. Not only will your metabolism speed up, but your body will work more productively and faster. Fasting takes digestion off your body's to-do list and allows your cells to rejuvenate and heal. When you are fasting, your body starts to produce stem cells - stem cells provide new cells for your body and replace cells that are damaged. Fasting is one of the best ways to detox your body fully and detox comes to many other great benefits, such as clear skin, balanced pH, better digestive health, boosted immune system, improved liver function, and more energy. Deciding to reboot your body is one of the best decisions you can make and the next doctor's appointment, after introducing intermittent fasting into your life, will be much more different than the previous ones.

The top 10 global causes of death include heart diseases, stroke, diabetes, and kidney failures. Interestingly enough, it is proven that intermittent fasting can improve all of these and change your life, without having to start your day with 5 pills in the morning, just to be able to live a normal or better life. Some people are not interested in losing weight and it is important to remember that intermittent fasting is not all about weight loss, it is not a weight-loss trend, even if some people may look at it like that.

It is clear that intermittent fasting can improve our health, but some of the benefits can help us live a longer and healthier life, by preventing serious health conditions.

Diabetes

Some people refer to diabetes as the biggest epidemic of the twenty-first century.

According to the World Health Organization (WHO), and the data on *Diabetes*, the number of people with diabetes rose from 108 million in 1980, to 422 million in 2014. More than

1.9 billion people are overweight and about 312 million of them are obese. Almost all diabetic people are overweight and that is because obesity causes increased levels of fatty acids,

leading to insulin resistance. Each year, there are about 7 million people that develop diabetes, mostly developing type-two diabetes and that is a very concerning number, to say the least.

Diabetes is also a major cause of blindness, kidney failure, and heart attacks (2020). Evidence has shown that fasting is an effective treatment for type 2 diabetes, it can help you manage your blood sugar, lower insulin levels and lose weight. Dansinger. M (2020) a dietary expert, did a shocking review in a recent study - people that have been struggling with type-two diabetes, for 10-25 years, were able to stop taking insulin within just a month, after fasting for 3 days a week or fasting every other day. In other studies, people with type-one diabetes (which is

insulin-dependent diabetes, because their bodies produce little to no insulin at all and apparently have no cure) were able to lower their insulin doses, after practicing intermittent fasting.

Heart disease

Many studies have found that people who practiced intermittent fasting for 6-24 weeks, were able to lower their blood pressure and it was not just explained by the weight loss. The American Heart Association has reported that intermittent fasting is associated with lower rates of heart failure and a longer life span, as well as causing a significant change in blood cholesterol levels and the outcome of these studies was unexpected, mentioning that long-term fasting can be extremely beneficial to our heart and overall health. There are several mechanisms for how fasting can lead to better cardiovascular health, some of them being the oxidative stress hypothesis, circadian rhythm hypothesis, and ketosis. Ketosis itself may have several health benefits, such as reduced seizures in children with epilepsy. So why are doctors not suggesting intermittent fasting as a non-medical treatment for people with diabetes and heart diseases? While some doctors are still skeptical due to unknown reasons, more and more doctors have seen major changes in their patients and therefore, they have started advising to include intermittent fasting into their patients' lives for weight loss and other health improvements. Not to mention that many doctors and physicians nowadays are practicing intermittent fasting themselves, after many studies and researches that have proven how fasting can impact our lives in a major way, as well as seeing great changes in their patients' health improvement.

Oxidative stress

While it sounds difficult, it is very simple. Your body produces free radicals during healthy and normal metabolic processes. However, oxidative stress means that there are more free radicals in your cells than needed. This can make you age quicker, damage your cells, DNA and proteins. Oxidative stress can be caused by different things, but some of them are your lifestyle and diet choices, health conditions, and other factors such as pollution and radiation. So how is this in any way related to intermittent fasting? Well, you guessed it. It has been proven that intermittent fasting can reduce oxidative stress, which means that it would benefit how you age and would prevent the development of certain diseases. A study on *Impact of Ramadan Intermittent Fasting on Oxidative Stress Measured by Urinary Isoprostane*, Al-Islam, M. et.al (2012), examined the impact of intermittent fasting on oxidative stress during Ramadan and found that the oxidative stress was in fact reduced, caused by weight loss. There was a major decrease in body fat and rapid weight loss is known to change circulating levels of oxidative stress markers.

Inflammation

Our bodies are extremely smart, our bodies protect us from viruses and bacteria twenty-four-seven, 365 days a year. Inflammation is a body's natural response to something that

is trying to damage your body and cells and you may notice redness, swelling, or even loss of function. Inflammation can also cause symptoms like fatigue, headaches, fever, and chills. Since intermittent fasting will help you with controlling your blood sugars, manage stress and make you lose weight, it will help you to reduce inflammation. Interestingly enough, inflammation also leads to serious health problems and diseases such as diabetes, multiple sclerosis, inflammatory bowel syndrome, arthritis, asthma, and even Alzheimer's disease. As you may notice by now, all of these health issues mentioned previously, go hand-in-hand with each other and one can lead to another and it truly does sound scary. There is a huge variety of medication to help with inflammation, but if we started taking pills for every small health-related issue that arises during our lives, all of a sudden it makes everything sound depressing, it is almost like our lives rotate around that and that only. Intermittent fasting is an easy way out when it comes to improving our general health and reducing inflammation - some studies show that intermittent fasting is one of the best non-medical treatments to help you reduce it.

Cancer

Cancer is the second leading cause of death, worldwide. It is a global burden. We all have family and/or friends that have either lived through the traumatic experience and have

fought cancer themselves, died of cancer, or were directly affected by it - losing family members and close people around them. Cancer can take a financial, emotional, and physical strain on families, individuals, and health systems. Usual survival rates are measured in a five-year survival rate. Let me repeat it - five years. While many people may take treatment well and live for longer, the average statistics are very sad. There are more than 100 types of cancer, including breast cancer, colorectal cancer, melanoma, bladder cancer, kidney cancer, lymphoma, lung cancer, and many more. Cancerous cells spread and grow incredibly fast, they can start spreading in any organ and spread to other organs, this process is called metastasizing. In metastasis, the cancerous cells break away from the original tumor, travel through the lymph and blood system, and form a new tumor. Once this process has started, there is almost no way to stop it and it is considered stage-four cancer and is terminal. There are promising cancer treatments like chemotherapy, radiation therapy, immunotherapy, hormone therapy, targeted therapy, and stem cell transplant. So where does intermittent fasting come into the picture, you may ask? Considering the fact that intermittent fasting causes several beneficial effects on metabolism, that may lead to a reduced risk of cancer. Also, evidence shows that intermittent fasting can reduce the bad side effects of chemotherapy, including tiredness and feeling sick. It is true that more human studies are needed, yet evidence shows that intermittent fasting can help prevent the risk of cancer in animal studies and decrease cancer growth rates.

Different studies state that intermittent fasting can increase the production of tumor-killing cells, trigger stem cells to regenerate the immune system and all types of cancer affect the body's immune system.

In a study focusing on a fasting-mimicking diet promoting T Cell-mediated tumor cytotoxicity, Di Biase, S. et.al (2016), showed that intermittent fasting and chemotherapy combined, slowed the process progression of skin and breast cancer. The treatment caused the body to produce high levels of lymphoid progenitor cells (known as CLP's) and tumor-infiltrating lymphocytes that are known to migrate into a tumor and start attacking it.

It is clear that the health benefits that come with intermittent fasting are unbelievable. It is also good for your brain health - because of reduced oxidative stress, reduced inflammation, lower blood sugars, as well as insulin resistance. Fasting can also prevent Alzheimer's disease and for Alzheimer's disease, there is no known cure and it is the world's most common neurodegenerative disease. Intermittent fasting cannot cure it, but it can prevent it. The evidence says that a lifestyle, that includes intermittent fasting, can reduce the severity of it and may delay the onset of Alzheimer's disease. Considering how many studies, clinical trials, and researches have been done to understand the positive effects of intermittent fasting, means that there is a reason behind it and this reason is very, very simple. It works and it is definitely not just a myth. It makes all of us wonder - what would actually happen if everyone started fasting, right? Would it be a huge loss to the pharmacy business, would it make the world a better, healthier place? We will never know. But what we can do, right now, is to re-think our lifestyle, our habits, our diets, and where our current health is at. We can take matters into our hands and prevent us from the risk of developing diabetes, cancer, and other terrible diseases.

"Therapeutic fasting is not a mystical or magical cure. It works because the body has within it the capacity to heal when the obstacles to healing are removed. Health is the normal state.

Most chronic disease is the inevitable consequence of living a lifestyle that places disease-causing stressors on the human organism. Fasting gives the body an interlude without

those stressors so that it can speedily repair or accomplish healing that could not otherwise occur in the feeding state." (Fuhrman, cited in Fasting and Eating for Health 1995)

Here's what you need to know

While fasting may sound like it is very easy to practice, there are many things you need to keep in mind and make sure you do it the right way, to lose weight and gain all the health benefits fasting can provide. The beginning is hard when it comes to everything and everyone and intermittent fasting will not be an exception, as long as you do it for the right reason and you have a certain goal. If you are new to intermittent fasting, you need to get into it by taking one step at a time, so jumping into three-day water fast may not be the best idea unless you are getting married in three days and you suddenly realize that your dress is not fitting you that well anymore, but that is a story for another day. You need to have an adjustment period, even if you want to lose as much weight as you possibly can, quickly. So how do you do it, how do you prepare your body for this huge change and how do you prepare yourself?

Write your goals on a piece of paper

Sit down and think about the main reason why you want to introduce intermittent fasting into your life, think about the reason behind all the reasons you can possibly come up with. Thinking about your weight and health goals can be easily compared to wealth goals. Everyone wants to be wealthy, but many people cannot give a proper reason why. When you have someone that says: "I want to be rich!" and you ask them - why? They usually would say something along the lines of "I want to buy my dream car or my dream house" and if you ask them the same thing again - but why? They usually get stuck. They cannot come up with an answer. Why do you want a big, beautiful house? Do you want to raise your children there and give them the life that you did not have? Do you want people to think that you have "made it"? Do you want to sleep in a different room every night? Why? You have to have an answer to these follow-up questions, even if no one is probably going to ask them. Do you want to start fasting to live a longer life?

Do you want to start fasting, because you have struggled with your weight for your whole life and it is making you absolutely miserable? Do you want to have a better quality of life? Write these things down and think about it before you are ready to jump into it because fasting is certainly a lifestyle and not a diet.

Prepare the people around you

As much as you wish, not everyone is going to understand your new lifestyle choices. Some might even be concerned and tell you that you are going to damage your health and you are going to starve yourself and this is just a trend that everyone has been following, but you should not. Is it your job to educate them? Well, if you feel like it. But it is possible that they still may not understand, so it really depends on you. Are you doing this for yourself or other people?

Imagine yourself in a year - if you took their advice and went back to the comfort of food and eating three to six meals a day, are you going to feel better, are you going to be healthier? And then imagine yourself in a year if you listened to yourself. Ironically, the same people that told you that you are starving yourself are the first people to congratulate you on your weight loss and tell you how beautiful you look. You do not have to make your family or the people around you do the same thing, but you should let them know that nothing is going to change in the family dynamics, but the time you eat - that's it. Do not be scared to tell people about you trying to live a healthier lifestyle, but remember that simply not everyone is going to understand it the right way. Be open about it and you also may inspire your family members, friends, and co-workers to do the same, once they start seeing the positive change in you. Next thing you know, you will be someone's body goals, you will be someone's wellness coach without being a wellness coach and people will look up to you. If you want to start seeing the results for yourself first, without telling anyone, or you may doubt intermittent fasting in general or doubt yourself and that you can do this and stick to your own promises, that is also fine - just remember the main reason why you are doing this.

Do not make bad decisions

Whether you choose to eat one meal a day or eat within a four-hour eating window, do not make unhealthy food choices, just because you have this amazing idea of losing weight, because you are fasting for a long period of time. Your body cannot do all the job for you and while you can eat your favorite foods within your eating window, that does not necessarily mean that you can consume fast food and fast food only. Not only intermittent fasting will not work, but you may feel even worse afterward. Feel free to have potatoes, tacos, and a cake when you really want it, do not restrict yourself - you can have it. But also include healthy fats like avocado, peanut butter, nuts, olives, and fish into your diet. Include lean meats, dairy products, and eggs into your diet. Have some variety on your plate and make it look beautiful, that way you will enjoy the food you are eating way more. It is okay if you are not the biggest fan of vegetables, you can easily change the way you consume them. Add some spinach and greens in your banana-strawberry smoothies and you will never be able to tell it is there. Add some bell pepper, tomatoes, and spinach to your pizza, and top it up with the stuff you like.

Add broccoli or cauliflower to your mashed potatoes and you will be amazed by the taste it will give your food, even if you absolutely hate broccoli and cauliflower. Enjoy your food and be creative with it, take your time to eat it, learn to understand what each thing on your plate means to your health and well-being.

Make your meals beautifully, decorate your plate, make it look like art and you will never look at the foods you used to eat - the same.

Choose the right plan for yourself

Okay, you have seen and read the reviews. People that eat one meal a day or fast for 72 hours have had amazing results and you want to have the same kind of results, I totally understand. But do not jump into it by choosing the most difficult intermittent fasting method right away. You will learn about the most effective fasting methods as you keep on reading, but you have to prepare yourself. Start with cutting out sugar and cream and drink your morning coffee plain.

Drink more water than you usually do in the mornings, as soon as you wake up. Take your time to drink your coffee and try not to focus on what you will be having for breakfast, eat it 2-3 hours later than you usually would. Try to have a nutritious dinner and do not go for a snack before going to sleep. These little-by-little steps will prepare you and will challenge you in a way as well. You will notice that you are getting super hungry in the morning, as you normally would have had your breakfast by now, but take notes on how you deal with it and how you are able to overcome the hunger, by drinking more water, for example. Pay attention to how you are able to focus better and how your mind works, while in a fasting state. Challenge yourself to let your body rest after dinner and go to sleep early, do not let the boredom fool you, because you know you are not hungry. Drink some green tea about 2 hours before going to bed, as it will help you sleep better and reduce stress. Try different fasting methods, if you feel like the first option you chose is not working for you, or you notice major changes in your mood swings, irritability, how your brain functions, or maybe you have been craving more carbs than ever and it is making you fail and give up completely. You have the freedom to change the timing, the foods you are consuming, you can add supplements or remove them from your diet, you can explore the internet and try new recipes, you can try making your first Keto cake with almond or coconut flour, instead of the usual white flour and see how you like it if you are a big cake lover or you love baking. There are many options and it can suit your lifestyle and food preferences the way no other diet or weight loss method can.

Overeating and not eating enough

Not eating enough can make you gain weight. Crazy, right? It is very, very real. When you are not consuming enough calories, your body starts to panic, because it does not get all the nutrients that it needs and your metabolism can slow down, meaning you can actually start gaining weight. In the same way, obesity is a huge global issue, under-eating is just as big of a problem and can lead to very bad things. Some people eat less than they should because of stress, chronic dieting, a restricted diet, or simply because they might be too busy. While they may seem healthy and fit from the outside, the consequences are terrible - their blood sugars are on a roller coaster, meaning they could experience anxiety, dizziness, shakiness, weakness, confusion, major mood swings, and sweating.

Some women are unable to get pregnant, due to hypothalamic amenorrhea - hallmarked by menstrual irregularity. Hypothalamic amenorrhea is caused by poor nutrition and extreme caloric deficit. Some people may be totally unpredictable because they might be hungry but are terrified of gaining weight and that is where the term hangry comes into the picture and it is not just a myth. Some people may experience sleep issues, insomnia, or other sleep disturbances, and is very common in people that do not consume enough calories and nutrients. The worst thing someone could do is under-eat and over-exercise, their liver will not have the glycogen stores it needs to keep their blood sugar stable.

The same goes for over-eating, you cannot consume 4000 calories a day and expect great results, even if you are fasting, your body simply cannot take that much and it can be extremely harmful to your health. How many calories a person should consume depends on each person individually, a bodybuilder can consume up to 3800 calories per day during their bulking phase, but these people also work out up to 4 hours a day and are burning many calories during this period. Try to be mindful with your food and do not put pressure on your digestive system, whether fasting or not. Overeating can cause your stomach to expand beyond its normal size to adjust the large food intake and that can damage other organs, making you very uncomfortable.

If you overeat all the time, or even with every meal you have, your digestive process will be slowed down and the food you consume will most likely be in your stomach for a longer time and it will most likely turn into fat. If we go into depth with this, medically, here is what happens.

If you eat past the point when you are feeling full, the esophagus fills with extra acid, resulting in heartburn. Your heart also speeds up as your metabolism increases to digest all the food. Your liver and pancreas start working harder to secrete extra hormones and enzymes to break down the food you have consumed. By overeating and gaining excess fat, you can increase the risk of developing cancer.

Intermittent fasting and exercise

There is some controversy around fasting and working out. There are many pros and cons, but what is the reality?

The thing is, working out will never hurt anyone. But if you are fasting, you have to be careful and you have to know how to combine the two, in order to achieve results. You can be burning more fat, especially if you work out while in a fasting state, but you also may not be able to build muscle and you may not have as much energy to work out in the first place.

A study on *Effects of aerobic exercise performed in fasted v. fed state on fat and carbohydrate metabolism in adults: A systematic review and meta-analysis* by Cambridge University (2016), found that that low-to-moderate intensity exercise performed in a fasted state can help you burn more fat, compared to exercise followed by eating a carb-containing meal.

Federation of American Societies for Experimental Biology (FASEB) found that exercise combined with fasting can trigger metabolic effects and improve muscle performance (2016). So... to workout or not to work out, that is the question. And the answer is pretty simple - listen to your body. Start with low-intensity workouts and see how you feel, see if you start having different cravings, see how well you perform during these workouts, and see if there is any difference in weight gain/loss and continue doing what works for you. If you are used to

high-intensity workouts, you may want to change your workout routine and adjust it, so you gain all the perks from working out and fasting at the same time. The best fasting workouts are jogging, cycling, doing yoga, and pilates. Weight lifting may not be the best option, so you should stick to cardio mostly. It is important to remember about protein after your workout, so it is advisable to work out while you are in a fasting state and then consume protein, healthy fats, and carbs high in fiber, you can also have a protein shake, to achieve better results.

Clean fasting and dirty fasting, what does that even mean?

During your fast, you should not have anything that could spike your insulin levels. You can stay away from food all day and all night, but you can have something so simple as sugar-free chewing gum, and oops, you are not fasting anymore. You can stay away from food, but take your daily vitamins and again, you are not fasting anymore. You can add berries and peppermint leaves to your water and it does not mean that you need to eat them, to break your fast, just having them in your water will break your fast alone. Even herbal tea has a huge question mark on it, as it can easily spike your insulin and your fast is done just like that. Is that considered dirty fasting though? Not really. People who "dirty fast" would even take the extra step and add milk or cream to their coffee or have up to 100 calories during fasting. This is something that you should not consider, as it will not give you the results you want even twice as fast, it will slow down the whole process and honestly, beat the purpose of fasting. You can drink black, unsweetened coffee, green unsweetened tea, mineral water, electrolytes, and salt in your water can be added as well and you will be in a clean fasting state. Even brushing your teeth can break your fast, if it contains sweeteners such as xylitol. They do not contain any calories, but this alone can cause an insulin spike, so be very careful when it comes to swallowing toothpaste. You definitely should not stay away from brushing your teeth or brushing your teeth during your eating window, but be careful. Interestingly enough, some people actually say that brushing their teeth while they are really hungry, during their fast, can help reduce the hunger pains and make you forget about wanting food.

What to eat during a feeding window - the key nutrients for intermittent fasting

The benefits of intermittent fasting are not likely to accompany consistent junk-food meals. What you consume during your feeding window will show in your progress, especially if your main goal is to lose weight. A well-balanced diet is a key and you should still focus on nutrient-dense foods, unprocessed and high-fiber foods, like vegetables, fruit, lean meats, healthy fats, dairy, proteins, whole grains, nuts, beans, and seeds. But let us start with the most important part - **water**. First, water will help you get through intermittent fasting because there might and most likely will be days where you feel like giving up and just stuffing your face with whatever, whenever. Water will help you to reduce hunger pains and make you feel fuller, as well as give you the hydration that you need, during the fasting state. Avoiding this part of the fast makes zero sense, as water is very important for our organ well-being in general, even without intermittent fasting. The amount of water you should drink depends on your body type, activity level, height, weight, and even climate, but an adequate daily water intake is about 2 - 3 liters per day, for both men and women.

If you are a **coffee** lover - this one is for you. But keep in mind, you may have to switch up a thing or two because if you love a really sweet frappé, iced caramel mocha latte, coffee milkshakes, or any other sweet coffee drinks, it will not be the best option. Although, if you stick to the main intermittent fasting rules and have a sweet coffee drink during your eating window, it is alright, do not make that an everyday thing, as it can slow down the whole process. The best thing to have is plain, unsweetened coffee without any sweeteners or milk added. Plain coffee can help you burn fat on itself and has many health benefits apart from intermittent fasting, so it is highly advised to include coffee in your diet. Coffee can be consumed during the fasting state as well and can be another secret weapon of staying on track, just like water.

In short, any drink that contains calories will break your fast. But there is one more thing you can have, without having to worry about breaking your fast and that is **green tea**. Herbal, detox, iced teas and anything that could contain calories should be avoided at all costs, as it can break your fast without even you knowing. Just like coffee and water, green tea also can help you with fat loss and has many health benefits, including improved brain function, may protect your brain from aging, reduce bad breath and possibly help with preventing cardiovascular diseases. You can have as much unsweetened green tea as you like, both during your fasting state and your feeding window.

If you plan on starting a fast, you may want to go through your pantry and your refrigerator, remove anything that may distract you from staying on track and simply go grocery shopping, get healthy, nutritious things that will motivate you and will make you feel better and improve your fasting experience. Your grocery shopping list should include **proteins**, like tuna, salmon, cod, shrimp, prawns, scallops, tilapia, turkey breast, trout, mussels, chicken breast, ground turkey, tofu, egg whites, walnuts, peanut butter, cashews, walnuts, and coconut. **Vegetables** like artichoke, broccoli, cauliflower, cabbage, beans, kale, greens, spinach, sweet potatoes, brussel sprouts, carrots, squash, lentils, peas, onions, shallots, garlic, beets, lemongrass, radishes, okra, cucumbers, eggplant, tomatoes, zucchini, peppers. **Fruit** like apples, melon, papaya, lemon, raspberries, strawberries, blueberries, figs, pear, dates, oranges, plums, grapefruits, nectarines, grapes, mango, pineapple. **Grains** like bulgur, buckwheat, oats, quinoa, rice, spelt, chickpeas, freekeh, whole-wheat couscous, corn. **Dairy** products like unsweetened almond, rice or soy milk, greek yogurt, cottage cheese, low-fat cheese, plain cream cheese. **Condiments** like any kind of vinegar, soy sauce, ketchup or tomato paste, hot sauce, sriracha, pesto, low sodium broth, fat-free cooking spray, herb paste, any kind of mustard, reduced-sodium teriyaki.

Supplements can be a part of your daily routine, but it is important to know when to take them. If your supplements contain any calories, avoid them during your fasting period and take them during your eating window. Some of the best supplements include electrolytes, probiotics, omega-3 fatty acids, chromium, amino acids, magnesium, zinc, protein powders, fat-soluble vitamins, fish oil.

What you should not be eating if practicing intermittent fasting is the type of stuff you would want to avoid even when not fasting - fast food. The main idea here is, you can eat it, but you really want to avoid it. If you crave a burger, do not hesitate to have the burger, but do not make that a daily habit and try to stay away from processed foods and foods that are high in carbs, as it may make you crave carbs even more than usual, during your fasting state. Sugary sodas and sweetened fruit juices. (for some reason, if we think about any movie that has a breakfast scene, fruit juice seems like a must-have, but you really want to avoid these - the more concentrated sugar, the more calories, the bigger chance for you to gain weight)

What does science say?

There is credible science and evidence for the benefits of fasting. Intermittent fasting was one of the most searched diets in 2019, although, let us not look at it as a diet, but as a way of life.

There are many evidence-based facts and some of them are the change of cell, hormone, and gene functions, reduced body fat, reduced insulin resistance, lower risk of developing diabetes, reduced oxidative stress and inflammation, improve numerous heart disease risk factors, cellular repair processes, cancer prevention, improved brain function and last but not least, a longer lifespan. Ramadan is a great example - millions of Muslims fast every day during the month of Ramadan, from dawn to sunset. Muslims are obligated to abstain from eating and drinking, including water. Mosques would provide iftar (morning meals, after fasting) to come together and to end the fast together. For Muslims, this is a spiritual cleanse, more than anything else. Many types of research have focused on what happens before, during, and after Ramadan, when people stop fasting and it has been proven that the overall health of people that always fast during Ramadan are generally healthy, and that definitely says something about fasting. It proves that the health benefits are nowhere near a myth. When you Google search "science and losing weight" the very first thing to be on the list is intermittent fasting, only then comes tracking your diet and exercise, cutting back on sugar, eating mindfully… So how come people, even some doctors, and health physicians are still so skeptical, when it has clearly been proven that intermittent fasting is not just a quick fix, not a trend, and not one of those crash diets that will make you gain even more weight? The truth is, there are many articles, many interviews with doctors, and many opinions, stating that intermittent fasting can actually damage your health, you should not try it, it is too extreme, but there is not a single study, a clinical trial, or research that has the evidence to prove these health risks scientifically and the outcome of each one of these studies are similar - reduced weight reduced blood pressure, reduced blood sugar. Health and excessive weight is something that everyone should take seriously and remember that a blog article is just a blog article and science is science. It is true that there are people who should not fast - people who struggle with an eating disorder should not try intermittent fasting, as it may resemble eating disorder behavior and can be a trigger for people who suffer from bulimia, for example. Pregnant women have been advised to stay away from fasting (especially during the time from week 22 to week 27) as well as women who are still breastfeeding, as it could be potentially harmful, but not in all cases. *The Journal of Nutrition* has published a study, by Tith. R. et.al. (2019) focusing on Fasting during Ramadan among Arabic-Speaking women which evaluated the association between fasting during Ramadan during pregnancy and it stated that the impact of fasting on the risk of preterm (which has been mentioned as the biggest concern by ob-gyn's) birth during Ramadan is unclear. They analyzed birth certificates from 3,123,508 child deliveries in Quebec, Canada, from 1981 to 2017 and focused on identifying Arabic-speakers among these birth certificates and determined if Ramadan occurred during the pregnancy.

They calculated the rates of preterm birth (late, very, and extreme preterm birth) and associated it with the results, stating that there were 215,317 preterm births out of 3,123,508 live births (6.9%) between 1981 and 2017, simply considering the fact that Arabic was the maternal mother-tongue, yet it is unclear whether these women were actually fasting during the month of Ramadan, so the result can be considered more assumption-based. Also, the same study shows that Arabic speakers had a lower rate of preterm birth compared with speakers of French, English, or other languages in Canada, where the study took place, it does not prove that women who fast during their pregnancy are in a greater risk of preterm birth.

According to Mattson. M and the neurobiological perspective, fasting can result in increased production of Brain-Derived Neurotrophic Factor (BDNF) signaling may meditate beneficial effects of fasting on glucose regulation and cardiovascular function. A review by Patterson and Sears (2017) on *The Metabolic effects of intermittent fasting*, states that eating patterns that reduce or eliminate night-time eating and prolong nightly fasting intervals may result in sustained improvements in human health.

Intermittent fasting regimens are hypothesized to influence metabolic regulation via effects on (*a*) circadian biology, (*b*) the gut microbiome, and (*c*) modifiable lifestyle behaviors, such as sleep.

A pilot study was done by the Department of Aging and Geriatric Research et.al (2019) reviewed the effects of intermittent fasting in older adults. Ten older overweight, sedentary adults of 65 and older, participated in this study and were fasting for 16 hours per day, for 4 weeks. The outcome of this study was amazing - in one month, there was noticeable body weight change, cognitive and physical function, lowered blood pressure and blood glucose. Also, these elderly participants had a small, but meaningful increase in walking speed on a 6-minute walking test that was done before and after the trial, and generally, walking speed is a strong predictor of major health outcomes in older adults.

In conclusion, the evidence-based facts and the science behind intermittent fasting and the major, not only health benefits but also life-improvement benefits are strong. If people around the world knew the facts, the benefits, and the truth behind this amazing power tool called fasting, high obesity, heart disease, and diabetes statistics would be drastically decreased.

While it may sound beautiful, the reality is and always will be different, but you have the opportunity to improve your health starting from today and that is the most important thing.

The best methods: How to choose the right one?

There are many ways you can include intermittent fasting in your life. In order to achieve the best results, you may have to try several methods and see what works for you the best.

What works for other people, may not work for you, more especially when we are talking about fat loss. However, the health benefits are still going to be there, no matter which method you decide to try.

The 12:12 method:

Simply the best method for beginners that want to introduce fasting into their lifestyle. This means that you eat for 12 hours and then fast for the next 12 hours. Experts say that the first results with this method will be visible in about 10 weeks and it is still possible to lose a lot of weight, even if the fasting window is not that big if you follow the routine and stick to your plan. After 12 hours, the food you have consumed has digested fully, which means that the next meal you consume is kind of like a fresh start. You should start easy, by having a light meal, to "wake up" your digestive system and this goes for all intermittent fasting methods, but it is just as important for the eat-stop-eat method since your body has digested all the food from your previous meals and you do not want to give your body a shock by eating a high-calorie meal, like a burger. Once you are able to go for 12 hours of not eating, try to go for 2 more hours because this is when your body is using your stored fat for energy and that happens after 14 hours. Once you are able to go without food for 14 hours, try going for 16 hours, but take your time and do not rush. Some days it may be harder and you may go from 16 hours back to 12 hours and that is okay, it happens and you should not beat yourself up about it, just know that tomorrow will be a better day.

The 16:8 method:

One of the most popular methods amongst people who practice intermittent fasting. There is an 8-hour eating window, then you fast for 16 hours. The 16:8 method can be a part of your everyday life and will lead to amazing results, with minimal effort. Here is an example of how you can do it: Skip breakfast. Drink water, black coffee without added sugar and cream, as well as green tea without added sugar. Have your first meal around 12 PM and eat as you normally would, without restricting yourself. If you want to achieve faster and better results, restrict your carbs and include healthy fats and protein. You can have as many meals as you want during these 8 hours, however, we suggest sticking to two - lunch and dinner, with a snack in between, if needed. Have your dinner before 8 PM and after that, you can still have water, tea, and coffee, but you should not be consuming any more calories. However, you can adjust the schedule as much as you like, as long as you follow these simple rules. It is proven that the 16:8 method boosts your brain function, and prevents diseases like diabetes and cancer. The results with this method will differ from a person to person, but the 16:8 has been found to be very effective - you can lose up to 20-30 pounds in a month and the nicest thing about this, is the fact that you do not need to change your life in a drastic way, just be patient until your next meal and enjoy the meals you have during those 8 hours.

The 5:2 method:

By choosing the 5:2 method, you will eat as you normally would for 5 days and then restrict your calories during the other two days. During these two days, the maximum calorie intake should not go over 500-600. The schedule is flexible, as long as there are two calorie-deficit days.

Eating 500 calories a day may sound scary, but you can still enjoy food and not feel hungry. Include vegetables, yogurt without added sugars, (greek yogurt, for example) lean meat, boiled eggs, greens, light vegetable soups. Include drinks like black coffee, green tea, and of course water. It is crucial to stay hydrated and drink plenty of water. The 5:2 method is extremely effective when done the right way and it's mainly because of the calorie deficit. A calorie deficit occurs when you consume fewer calories than you should, to maintain your weight.

The Warrior Diet:

The Warrior diet lives up to its name. This method is extremely effective for fast and sustainable weight loss and while it may seem similar to other intermittent fasting methods, the Warrior diet is known as one of the most effective ways to lose fat. This method is also called the 20:4 diet - however, the idea here is different. The Warrior diet includes restricting some foods for 20 hours and lets you eat as you wish, during a 4-hour eating window. During the first part of the day, you should eat very small portions of vegetables and raw fruit. During this phase, you should only drink water, black coffee, and green tea, without any added sugars. When it comes to dinner, for example, you can consume heavier foods and have a large meal. It is proven that people who followed the 20:4 method were able to lose more weight, than people who consumed the same amount of calories throughout the day. The Warrior Diet has been suggested by many doctors, researchers, and health experts, that truly believe that this method is one of the best intermittent fasting methods you can choose from, it is very sustainable and easy to follow. You will be extremely focused and alert during the fasting state And then get to feast and reward yourself with a nice meal.

Eat-stop-Eat

This method is very straightforward. You fast for 2 days a week and then eat responsibly for the rest of the 5 days. For example, you eat as you normally would on Monday and Tuesday, then you fast for 24 hours, eat normally again on Thursday, fast for 24 hours, and then eat normally again on the weekend. This method in general helps you to cut down on calories that you are consuming throughout the week and it will help you to shrink your belly, so you will start getting fuller a lot quicker. There is no evidence to prove that the eat-stop-eat method is better than any other intermittent fasting methods, but many people tend to enjoy this type of fasting method, considering the fact that you still get to eat once a day, if you choose to eat breakfast, then you can have breakfast the next day as well and then go back to your normal eating schedule, so it is pretty flexible. For people that have a hard time dealing with hunger, this method might work better than any other method, because you only fast for 2 days a week.

OMAD (One Meal A day)

While just some people this method can sound like torture, OMAD is one of the easiest and simplest ways to fast. You fast for 23 hours and eat for one hour. During that one hour, you can have whatever you want, and it is advised to consume at least 1000 or 1200 calories during that one meal. You can have your meal, have coffee, soda, milk, whatever it is that you want to have, and then you can have a break, go for a walk or prepare a quick dessert. If you had a really healthy meal and the calories would not be enough for you to fast for 23 hours, you can go back and have a dessert or even the second portion or you can have a nice cup of bulletproof coffee - black coffee with butter in it. It is popular amongst fitness enthusiasts because it can give you ample energy and be a great source of fat and can be around 250 calories. So if you are feeling super full already and you cannot and do not want to eat anymore, do not push yourself, but consider drinking the bulletproof coffee, which will give you the daily calorie count you are looking for, or a fruit-berry smoothie with milk with MCT oil added. MCT oil is a highly concentrated source of medium-chain triglycerides and can be beneficial for your health. If you are extremely busy and have a lot going on in your life, eating one meal a day can save you time, money, resources, and energy. You do not need to worry about what are you going to have for breakfast, or about going to the grocery store and thinking of what to buy for the next week, because if you are eating once a day, you can plan your one meal for the next three to four days, so food does not go to waste - if you buy as much food as you usually would, most likely you will end up throwing it out. With OMAD, all you need to care about is what you're going to eat just once and you will realize that you have saved yourself a lot of time and money.

You should try to avoid eating the same or similar food every day. If you eat fish, quinoa, a salad, and a slice of cheesecake one day have chicken with rice and ice cream the next day - try to switch it up and not make it boring. If you are going out for lunch with your buddies and you decide to go for fries, a burger, chicken nuggets, and onion rings, try to include more vegetables the next day, have a fruit smoothie, have peanuts or walnuts, and add some healthy fats to your meal, like try cooking with coconut oil.

Alternate day fasting:

With this method, there are several ways to do it, but the main idea is to fast every other day. You eat what you want one day, then fast the other day. During this fasting day, in order to achieve better results, you should not be consuming any calories, so sticking to plain water, coffee and unsweetened tea is the best way to do it. Some people do consume up to 500 calories during their fasting days but you need to remember that this will take you longer to lose weight because you are consuming calories at the end of the day. Some people find alternate-day fasting to be easy because they are able to eat whatever they want one day and all they need to do is stay away from food the next day, but on the other hand, some people may find it extremely difficult due to the fact that you cannot consume any food at all. The fasting window is very long so it might be harder for people that are used to having at least one meal a day, but you should still try it and it might be the best option that works for you. The plan is simple - on the first day, eat whatever you would usually eat. On the second day, have plain coffee, water, unsweetened green tea, but try staying away from food. On the third day, have whatever you want, there is nothing specific that you should do as long as you stick to healthy and nutritious meals. One of the biggest obstacles when it comes to alternate-day fasting is hunger. Your body will tell you that you need to eat, You will definitely hear your stomach growl and you also may experience some tiredness, mood swings, or even a slight headache. If you learn how to ignore these signals that your body gives you and you are able to stay away from food, drink more water, you might notice that with time it gets a lot easier and on the fasting day, your body will be used to you not eating and it will become easier to stick to this protocol and lose weight.

Extended/prolonged fasting

When you fast for 36 hours and more, it is called extended, or prolonged fasting. You can set a goal to fast for 36, 48, or 72 hours, that way it will be easier to stay on track, rather than doing a 40 hour fast and a 56 hour fast, you need to have a specific goal and go for it. Of course, if you do a 50 hour fast and cannot do anymore, that is still an amazing achievement on its own. In short, you eat nothing for 36 or more hours and only drink water, plain coffee, or unsweetened green tea. Some people prefer drinking water only, (also called water fast) but you can still allow yourself to have coffee and tea. While it may sound like starvation, an extended fast has way more health benefits than you realize. Remember that by 24 hours you have entered ketosis and autophagy, so imagine the benefits if you fast for 36, 48, or 72 hours. Your body has turned into a fat-burning machine and your body is doing a spring cleaning, while you sleep, while you work, while you are reading a book. If you are used to fasting for 16 or 23 hours, then a 36-hour fast sounds like mission impossible, but this has a lot to do with how prepared you are mentally as well, you have to be in a certain mindset and focused on your goal and the benefits of this type of fast, to be able to do it. You will be surprised by how light you will start to feel and how energized you are, even though we have been told that food gives us energy, and we need it to keep it moving. If you are doing an extended fast, you do have to be very careful with working out, you should not be lifting weights in the gym, as you will simply lose lean body muscle and mass.

It is not advised to go longer than 72 hours unless you speak to your doctor - some people do this to lose weight quickly, before a medical surgery, but you have to do it under your doctor's supervision and not on your own. It is also important what you eat after an extended fast, to avoid getting sick - you have to break the fast correctly, or else you will not want to try this ever again. It is advised to drink water with apple cider vinegar, to introduce acid back into your system and it will help you prepare your stomach for food again. The best thing you could have after a long fast is bone broth. Bone broth is a rich source of nutrients and will help you replenish electrolytes. It will not break your fast completely yet, that is why it is advised to do things gradually - apple cider vinegar and water, then the broth about 5 minutes later, then wait about 20 more minutes before you have your meal. When you are ready to eat, do not go all-in with a heavy meal, you should still consider eating lighter foods first, heavier foods after. You may start with chicken, or fish, avocado, cooked green vegetables and only then have something like pasta, or a curry, or a cake, if you want to. If you eat that before preparing your body, you will find yourself feeling extremely sick and your gut will not be happy about this.

The key is to stay patient and understand that you will be able to eat your food the way you want it, just do it gradually and you will get there. If you were able to do a prolonged fast, you are going to be able to wait for another 20 minutes.

The bottom line is, no matter which method you decide to choose, be proud of yourself for wanting to change your life and not waiting for Monday, be proud of the fact that you are doing something to improve your health. What works for others may not work for you, but you have all the freedom to try out different methods and see what works for you, what makes you feel good, and what makes you lose weight. Do not watch the scale every day, simply buy an outfit you would absolutely love to wear, but you do not fit in right now and make it your goal to wear it in a month, take pictures and that will motivate you to stay on track after you look back at what you have been able to achieve.

Your perfect guide to incredible results

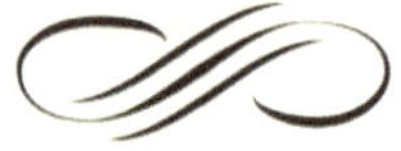

No more talking, it is time to take action. After you have talked to your family and made it known that you absolutely love the Sunday barbecue feasts, you love the weekly cake someone decides to bake, you love the high-carb breakfast with the kids in the morning before they leave for school, but you are not including yourself in each one of these feasts anymore and you have decided that it is time to change. It is time to surprise your doctor with the next check-up, time to make your co-workers jealous, and time to go on a shopping spree after none of your old clothes fit anymore.

Things that you need to get rid of

You went through your pantry and your refrigerator and understood what the main things you want to get rid of are, or what main things you will not want to include in your diet, like ready-to-eat meals that contain fake vitamins and minerals, that contain too many vegetable oils, too many chemicals (glycerin, sodium caseinate, artificial flavors) and are absolutely no good for anyone. You have found unhealthy condiments in your refrigerator, such as margarine, mayonnaise (unless you are doing Keto, try to make your own mayo), Ranch dressing (unless you need extra calories for your one or two meals a day, try to use Tahini sauce instead - it is made out of sesame seeds and although it is high in fat, it is good unsaturated fat), sour cream (use non-fat, plain greek yogurt instead), chocolate syrup that is super delicious, yet high in refined carbohydrates like fructose corn syrup (try eating dark, 80-90% cocoa chocolate from time to time, to satisfy the chocolate cravings, if you have any) and everyone's favorite - BBQ sauce, that is super high in sugar. Try making a homemade BBQ sauce, using pureed blueberries, mangoes, peaches, blackberries, agave syrup, unfiltered honey, and spices like paprika, cayenne pepper, red pepper flakes, cumin seeds, and vinegar.

A grocery shopping list for your new beginnings

Meat and fish: Chicken breast, ground beef, turkey, lobster, salmon, tuna, scallops, shrimp.

Vegetables: Broccoli, cauliflower, bell pepper, spinach, onion, zucchini, tomato, cucumber, radish, eggplant, garlic, lettuce, mushrooms, squash, green beans, cabbage, celery, sweet potato, corn, okra, pumpkin, leek, brussel sprouts, parsnip, peas, carrot, yam, beet, artichoke, asparagus, kohlrabi, fresh grape leaves, fresh coriander, fresh dill, arugula, kale, and microgreens.

Fruit: Strawberries, blueberries, cranberries, raspberries, blackberries, apple, avocado, grapefruit, jackfruit, grapes, coconut, lemon, pomegranate, kiwi, lime.

Plant-based proteins: Beans, lentils, tofu, hummus, vegetarian protein powder, chickpeas, peanuts, almonds, spirulina, quinoa, tempeh, edamame beans, chia seeds, hemp seeds, seitan Grains: Buckwheat, amaranth, brown, black or wild rice, barley, oats, spelt, bulgur, millet, farro, freekeh, fonio.

Dairy: Plain cottage cheese, plain greek yogurt, kefir, whey protein, eggs, low-fat cheese, or parmesan cheese.

Oils/fats: Walnut oil, coconut oil, avocado seed oil, grass-fed/organic butter, flaxseed oil, hemp seed oil, extra-virgin olive oil, low-sodium soy sauce, MCT oil, CBD oil.

Natural seasonings: Herbs, citrus, (freshly squeezed lemon or lemon pepper) sea salt/kosher salt, garlic, ground spices, shallots

Snacks: Granola bars, lentil chips, hummus chips, seaweed snack, rice cakes, low-sodium or vegetable pretzels, sunflower seeds, pumpkin seeds, low-fat string cheese, baby carrots, kale chips, organic chickpea snacks, olives, protein crackers, crispbread, apple chips, peach rings, berry-nut mixes, hard-boiled eggs, non-fat yogurt with fresh berries, guacamole with veggie pita crackers, fresh apple slices.

Beverages: Water, coconut water, ginger tea, green tea, herbal tea, freshly squeezed carrot juice (add a ½ tablespoon of extra-virgin olive oil or coconut oil, that will help you to absorb all the vitamins quicker) freshly squeezed green juice (with spinach, celery, kale, fresh ginger, lime juice, kiwi, apple), lemon-infused water, fresh beet juice, almond milk, rice milk, soy milk, plain coffee, organic matcha tea (matcha is a finely ground powder of specially grown green tea leaves and is high in antioxidants, protects the liver and also helps you lose weight) or kombucha (a fermented and sweetened black or green tea drink that contains good bacteria and yeast, consumed for health purposes)

Supplements: Creatine (creatine is an organic compound that increases your body's ability to produce energy rapidly), L-tyrosine (Tyrosine improves focus, alertness, and attention),

L-carnitine (Carnitine boosts your metabolism and can help you lose excess fat) electrolytes, (They are minerals that are vital for your nervous system and muscles), magnesium (another mineral that helps the nerves and muscles function properly), vitamin B, C, D, zinc and copper, protein powder (any kind of protein powder, as protein, is extremely important for weight loss) curcumin and green tea extract. (Can be taken in the form of pills)

Consider meal prepping

People tend to make unhealthy decisions when in rush, or when they are really hungry.

Considering that you will be fasting for a certain period of time, whichever method you choose, at some point, you will be famished and you will be ready to grab anything that looks good when your eating time has started. You may order a take-away, grab your car keys, and head to the closest fast-food place, grab all those healthy snacks mentioned previously and eat them all at once and end up overeating. Instead, consider preparing your meals for the next two or three days. You will be able to measure the nutrients and portion sizes, again, to avoid overeating when you are trying to break your fast. A collection of well-balanced meals, consumed at the right time, will help you stay on track and achieve your goals way faster. Not only that, but you will save time, money, energy, stress, calories, and even prevent food waste.

Start with preparing lunch for the next three days - prepare quinoa, (add spices and herbs to the hot water, let it sit, and let quinoa absorb the water) roast some vegetables in the oven, (broccoli, carrot, asparagus) take a chicken breast, season it with your favorite spices, add extra-virgin olive oil in the pan (you may use an oil/cooking spray, like a rosmarino spray) and cook until golden brown. Get three food containers and add equal portions of quinoa, roasted veggies, and chicken. Store them in the refrigerator and have a nice, healthy lunch ready to eat!

Healthy alternatives

If you noticed - sugar, pasta, lemonade, chocolate pudding, pancakes, fries, and ice cream has not been mentioned on the shopping list. But what do you do if you are a pasta lover if you absolutely cannot live without a chocolate pudding? Here is the trick - everything has a good alternative.

Eat guilt-free zoodles (zucchini noodles) instead of spaghetti. Add a homemade bolognese sauce with crushed tomatoes, fresh herbs, onion, garlic, and ground turkey.

Instead of lemonade or a cold soft drink, take peppermint leaves, slices of lemon, and lime and leave it all in a bottle of water, leave it in the refrigerator for an hour and enjoy a cold, healthy drink.

Instead of a ready pancake mix that is super high in all the wrong things, try protein pancakes. Take your favorite protein powder, eggs, a banana, oats, a bit of salt and cinnamon, and baking powder, mix it together and you have some delicious, healthy, light, and fluffy pancakes.

Forget about white rice - use brown, black, or wild rice instead. Or just use cauliflower rice - cut the cauliflower into larger chunks, place it in a food processor, or hand-grate the cauliflower until it looks like rice. Then sauté in a large skillet, add some fresh herbs, toasted almonds, finely diced tomatoes, jalapeño, and stir it all together.

Replace your favorite chocolate pudding with a chia seed pudding: Take chia seeds, plant-based milk like cashew or almond milk, maple syrup, add fresh fruit and mints.

Kale chips instead of potato chips - you can make them on your own. Simply wash some kale, put it on a baking sheet, add a few drops of olive oil, season the kale leaves, and put it in the oven. Or you can get seaweed snacks, there are sea salt seaweed snacks, wasabi seaweed snacks, even seaweed in tempura. (Seaweed in tempura will be higher in calories, but still can be an option if you crave something crunchy)

Bake a crust-free pizza, instead of ordering a large pepperoni pizza from your favorite pizza place. Take portobello mushrooms or slice zucchini in half, take the middle part out and stuff the mushrooms or the zucchini with olives, shredded chicken, mushrooms, bell pepper, chopped artichoke, and mozzarella cheese.

Create your own dip for your baby carrots, hummus chips, or crackers - a tomato salsa with tomatoes, onion, garlic, lime, and coriander, or make your own tzatziki sauce from scratch, using natural yogurt, garlic, mint leaves, cucumber, and lemon juice.

Make your own ice cream at home, by using greek yogurt, coconut milk, protein powder of your choice, dates, and a little bit of vanilla extract - mix it, freeze it, then enjoy your homemade,

low-calorie, healthy ice cream.

You are a huge cake lover? No problem. You can try making a homemade cake with honey, oat milk, coconut oil, sea salt, yeast, and eggs, mix it together, pour the mixture in a baking pan, top it with fruit, nuts, oats, and when ready, grate dark chocolate over it. Or make a chocolate zucchini cake (Yes, I know what you are thinking right now, but keep on reading) with zucchini, eggs, oat milk, unsweetened cocoa powder, dark chocolate, cinnamon, maple syrup, figs, and dates, add baking powder and mix it all together - you will love this recipe.

The before and after

We all have seen those super inspiring people that have lost a large amount of weight, do the before and after pictures - and we thought to ourselves: "I would love to be able to do the same!" Well, guess what - you are going to do it now. First, grab a pen and paper, a measurement tape, and the scales. Measure your bust, waist, hips, and thighs. Write it all down and then get on the scales. Measure your current weight and think about your goal weight, what is the number that you are looking for and you can use these abbreviations: SW (Starting weight); CW (Current weight); GW (Goal weight) as it will be easier for you to understand what is what. Find a family member, a friend, a colleague, a stranger on the street and ask them to take a few pictures of you, to compare your progress. Ideally, you can do it all in one notebook, have all the measurements and pictures in one place, it will be interesting for you to go back and look at it, once you have reached your goals. Do a weekly weigh-in and again, measure your bust, your waist, hips, and thighs, and keep doing it every week. The motivation you will gain from seeing the numbers becoming lower and your weight decreasing, will keep you going, although remember water weight exists and if every other day is not a cheat day for you, you have to keep going and understand that those fat cells will burst eventually.

Plan, plan, and plan some more

If you are an outgoing person, you have plenty of friends and family members - therefore, many birthdays, weddings, engagement parties, and baby showers. Since food is one of the main things everyone looks forward to, that does not mean that you cannot. If you decide to just skip breakfast and you are attending a birthday dinner at 7 PM, you are more than good to go. Since it is a birthday dinner, no one is going to get up from the table after they are done eating - usually, people eat and eat, non-stop, take a smoke break maybe, but then return to the

table filled with food, have great conversations with people around them and again, continue eating. What you can and should do is enjoy the dinner, enjoy food and a glass of wine until 9 PM, then have a cup of coffee with a birthday cake like everyone else and stop right there.

Usually, you would stop fasting around 8 PM, this time you have stopped around 10 PM and it is okay. But since the usual first meal of the day would be at 12 PM the next day, make it till 2 PM.

You will not faint during those two hours, just drink more water, get coffee or green tea, stay busy and you might even miss your feeding time because hunger does go away if you ignore it. If you want to go back to your normal 12 PM/8 PM schedule, simply stop eating at 8 PM, do not make it till 10 PM again. Have a nice, filling dinner that will keep you going until the next day's 12 PM. If you know that your family is going all out for Christmas and has started cooking 2 days prior, enjoy a full day of eating, then do a water fast the next day, to flush it all out and you can go back to your normal schedule. If you love leftovers the next day, fine - eat it once and forget that it exists, stay motivated, stay on track, do not make excuses for yourself, just because it is Christmas and there is delicious food right in front of you. Dedication is the key!

Let's talk Keto

It is possible that you have heard of this word before. You have heard about it at work, from your friends, from your family, but you are not sure what Keto means exactly. Or you have seen loud, attention-catching blog posts or social media posts that say: "Lose weight, now! Quickly! Tons of weight! Eat bacon and cheese and mayo and STILL LOSE WEIGHT" and you probably thought to yourself: "Another lie. Another misleading title, it would not work and I am not even going to try it." What if I told you that it does work? What if I told you that your body will burn fat, while you are eating bacon? Makes no sense, right? Here is how it works. Keto stands for ketosis or the ketogenic diet. A diet that tells you to eat fat, something completely different from what we have heard all of our lives - eat less fat. Even if it makes no sense, it does work.

People all around the world have jumped on it and have had incredible weight loss results. Results that are so quick and visible, that it could be compared to gastric bypass surgery, a surgery where the doctors would make your stomach smaller, so you are simply not able to consume large amounts of food and you are able to lose weight quickly and effectively. But how does Keto work then, if you are allowed to eat such fatty foods?

The ketogenic diet is against carbohydrates - all kinds of them. Good carbs, bad carbs, it does not matter. Even the healthiest things have carbs, some have less, some have more. But the idea behind this is that you should not consume more than 50g net carbs. The difference between these two is that from all the carbs that may contain sugar, fiber, and starches, you have to focus on the actual carbs (net carbs), that will turn into glucose and that is what you should be counting. But why carbs? Why is that even a worry?

We should be staying away from sugar, we all know that. But not everyone understands that carbs literally turn into sugar. You can eat rice, which does not remind you of sugar at all, but that turns into glucose (blood sugar) in your body and uses this glucose as a source of fuel. Normally, people that eat around 2000 calories a day, consume about 200-300 grams of carbs.

In the Keto language, 50 grams is too much already, that would be considered "dirty Keto". Ideally, a perfect Keto is 20 grams and below. In a normal world, eating rice, beans, plantain, and sweet potato is considered pretty healthy, but in the Keto world, the more fat, the more cheese, the more eggs, the better. Still not convinced? We can talk about science and biology. Once you stop consuming high amounts of carbs, your body enters ketosis - a metabolic state that you can achieve with intermittent fasting as well, for a short period of time, well, until you eat carbs again. With Keto, you never leave ketosis, which means once you have entered it and do not consume any carbs or sugar, your body burns fat and never really stops doing it. Once you have run out of glucose, your body still has to find some kind of energy source and becomes desperate. If glucose was used for it before, then now it has to be fat, meaning, you do not even need to work out and your body will be burning fat on its own. Not only that, but your brain can also use ketones for energy - your brain gets about 25% of its energy from the ketones if you are in ketosis or you are water fasting. If you are fasting for more than 72 hours, your brain uses 60% of its energy from ketones. But there are some things you need to consider before starting the keto diet. You have to know what to avoid and what can kick you out of ketosis, you have to understand what you should eat - usually, an app that counts macros would help you understand how many net carbs you are consuming in a day and will help you see if there is anything you need to adjust and change. With time, you will simply know what to eat and what not to eat, but we all have to start somewhere. Now, if you are wondering why Keto is even mentioned in a book about intermittent fasting, wonder no more. If you take fasting with all the amazing benefits that come with it, plus the fat loss, and then take keto, combine that together and all of a sudden, having that beach body does not sound far from reality, does it?

Here is how keto intermittent fasting would look like. You have your first meal at 12 PM, you have an omelet with cheddar cheese, bacon, and coffee with heavy cream. You decide to have a snack at 3 PM and you go for mozzarella cheese sticks (not fried) and guacamole. You make a big dinner for the whole family at 6 PM - you are grilling chicken, putting broccoli and asparagus in the oven, as well as a huge pizza, that is made with cauliflower crust and no one would even be able to tell the difference. You also go for a glass of red wine and a keto cheesecake. You tasted everything, you had the chicken, the vegetables, the pizza, the cake, the wine, and only consumed about 10 grams of net carbs. With what you ate during the day, you will not go over the 20 grams of carbohydrates, even if you wanted to. If the dinner was finished around 8 PM and you did not eat anything until 12 PM, that means you have been fasting for 16 hours and your body is in a full fat-burning state. Yes, even after a pizza, a cake, and a glass of wine, or two. The reason why keto is so popular, well, you probably understand by now. It is a simple diet that everyone can follow and still lose weight. Ketosis can have a few negative effects in the beginning, once you start living the full-on keto lifestyle, you may notice interesting things that may happen to you, and keto flu is one of them. Keto flu occurs when your body is adjusting to burning fat for energy, it can make you feel like you have the regular flu, with the typical flu symptoms - nausea, foggy brain, dizziness, muscle cramps and can last even for a week or more until your body is fully adjusted. You can try preventing it, but do not be scared of it, it is your body's natural response to you cutting out carbs. You can start adding more salt to your meals, increase electrolytes, drink plenty of water, drink bone broth with salt and spices in it.

While keto sounds very simple to follow, you do need to recognize when it is not for you and when you start damaging your health, without even knowing it. If you promise yourself to stay on track - with keto, you just have to do it. If you have a cheat meal while you are supposed to be fasting, it is okay - tomorrow will be a better day. With keto, if you have a cheat meal and eat something that is high in carbs, it will make you feel sick because your body will be extremely confused and you will not be in ketosis anymore. Without 24 hours of fasting straight, doing the keto alone will take you about a week to get back into ketosis. So, if you are doing great and after a month in, you decide to have pasta, you are out. You have to go back to not eating carbs for another week, just to be able to get into that metabolic state again, or else your body will not be burning any fat. Again, it is easy, but should be taken more seriously, as this can damage your health in the long run, especially if you have cheat meals like that every week and you never really get to the ketosis part. You end up eating high-fat foods while not being in ketosis, because you had carbs, meaning you are consuming way more calories than you need a day and you end up gaining weight.

It is common for beginners to make mistakes, so here are the most popular mistakes to avoid:

Be aware of hidden carbs

Just because you are avoiding things like bread, potatoes, and oats, does not mean that you are not consuming any carbs. Liquid eggs that come in a container are one of them - some people buy that just to make life easier, but please do not do that and buy real eggs. Liquid eggs contain egg whites with added beta carotene to make them yellow, they are nowhere near as nutritious as real eggs are - stick to the real deal. Peanut butter is great and should be added to your diet if you are not doing keto, but with keto, it is an absolute disaster, as 2 tablespoons of peanut butter contain about 6-7 grams of carbs and you will go way over the allowed limit of carbs easily. Sun-dried tomatoes might be a great addition to cauliflower rice dishes and your omelet, but 100 grams of sun-dried tomatoes alone go over your allowed daily carb intake, 23 grams of carbohydrates. You will have to say bye to beans as well - beans are healthy, yes. But keep in mind, that one gram of beans contains about 120 grams of carbohydrates and that is how much carbs you should consume in 6 days, that is a huge difference. Another important vegetable that should be in every diet, except keto, is corn. Corn on the cob, grilled corn, fried corn, forget about it. One cup of corn contains 41 grams of carbs, the yummy elote (a Mexican corn recipe) contains about 22 grams of carbs, that is what you should be consuming in a whole day. There are vegetables that are no-go for keto, especially root vegetables. What is so dangerous about them? Well, carbs. Many, many carbs. Beets, artichokes, carrots, cassava, squash, sweet potato, pumpkin, peas, yams - all of these vegetables contain about 13-30 grams of carbohydrates per vegetable. You can still have spinach that has zero carbs, celery that has 1 gram of carbs, as well as broccoli, cabbage, kale, cucumber, mushrooms, asparagus, lettuce, and peppers, they are safe and do not contain many carbs at all.

All you need to do is check nutrition labels, do your research on each individual vegetable, fruit, condiments, and other things that could potentially be high in carbs.

Too much, too little

Since keto is a diet that should be high in fat, you can easily go overboard and have too much dairy - not all forms of dairy are keto-friendly. Generally, keto should go like this - 70% of fat,

5-10% of carbohydrates, about 20% of protein. If you have too much protein, it will not kick you out of ketosis, but it can and will lower the ketones in your blood and you will not lose fat as quickly. If you do not eat enough fat, you may not even enter ketosis, you can even go higher and eat 80% of fat - sometimes it may feel like you are going to start gaining large amounts of weight by eating all that fat, but that is not how it happens with keto, you need the fat in your diet. Never go over the allowed percentage and not include any green vegetables in your diet, you should not be living off of bacon, eggs, and cheese alone. You will still lose weight, but that can impact your health badly, you need to include healthy options as well.

Another important piece of advice, get some proper sleep during the night. If you do not sleep long enough, or the quality of your sleep is not the best, your stress hormones will increase and that leads to high cortisol, which will make you gain weight. Sleep is important when it comes to any diet, so make sure you go to sleep at a decent time and get a good, quality sleep.

But how do you know when you are in ketosis? Apart from your body giving you many signals, you can measure how well you are doing. The most accurate way to check ketones is with a specialized meter, that measures ketones in your blood. You can test ketones in your breath, by using special devices, they check your ketone and acetone levels to tell you whether you are in ketosis or not. The third option is checking ketones in your urine, with urine test strips. They are reliable, however, checking your blood ketones is the most reliable way to do it.

Keto is a great way to achieve your weight loss goals without including intermittent fasting, but the sky's the limit here, combine the two and see how quickly your body adapts and how easily the weight comes off. If it does not work for you and you need carbs in your life, understandable - just stick to intermittent fasting, mindful eating, and healthier choices.

Lifestyle adjustments

To change your life, you have to change your mindset, master the mental game of becoming the best version of yourself. Every weight loss and health journey begins with a strong, determined mindset. If you stick to what you know, if you do not want to challenge yourself, you have a "maybe I am supposed to be this way" mentality, if you give up when you are frustrated, perhaps it is time to change your mindset. You have to understand that a challenge is an opportunity for you to grow, that you can do anything you put your mind to, that you are not going to fail this time. Many people struggle with their weight and while no one wants to be obese, unhealthy, and developing serious health conditions, there are not that many people who are ready to change their lifestyle, their habits and they choose acceptance over change the reality, but that does not mean you need to be one of them. It can be extremely hard to push yourself, and most probably, you have tried it before and it did not work, so why try again? It is possible that you have tried to do a crash diet and did not see any results, you have tried going to the gym, but felt like the odd one out, because there are a bunch of lean, fit, healthy people and you left without looking back. Maybe you struggle with emotional eating and food simply brings you comfort and you are not willing to give that up, at least not yet. But you have a choice. You have a choice to continue to live the same way, or a choice to say: "It is enough. I want to be healthy. I want to live an active, happy life."

Success does not come easy and it certainly will not be easy for you to not eat for 16 hours, all of a sudden. Starting somewhere will help you get used to it and you will start to mentally prepare yourself for the life ahead of you. You may do amazing in the first few days, you will be extremely excited to get on the scale and you may see that your weight has gone up. If you do not prepare yourself this mentally, you will get angry at yourself for even giving this a try and turn to something that makes you feel good, calms you down, and brings you comfort - and you guessed it. It is food. Once you are frustrated, it is possible that you will eat more than your stomach can even take. But why not, because nothing works anyway, right? No. This is not how this should and will work. You put the scale away, forget that you even own it, go and get a large bottle, fill it up with water, sit down and slowly drink it. With every sip you take, imagine the water making its way down to your system and visualize all the bad stuff exiting it. Water is pure, water is the main constituent of the earth's hydrosphere and is vital for all known forms of life and it is vital for you. Imagine all the toxins being flushed out, imagine the removed waste from your blood, all the benefits water can give you, and then think about the importance of it. When you have understood the importance of water, understand the importance of your organs, your digestive system, your heart most importantly. Excess fat tends to be all-around the most vital organs - the more fat you have, the less space for your organs to function properly. So when you are thinking of giving up and getting up to get another bag of chips out of frustration, because intermittent fasting is just another lie and a diet that could never work, think about how this and every next bag of chips will affect you. Try to see the bigger picture and do not focus on the fact that this one or a few bags of chips will not make a huge difference. It will and you do not need to wait until it damages your health to the point where you are unable to take care of yourself and be able to even get up and get that bag of chips.

Make sure to set goals. Set realistic goals. Every project, every business plan, every goal requires an action plan and you need to create one as well. A good intermittent fasting schedule has good planning and dedication behind it. Recognize and acknowledge your current issues and your bad habits. Whether it is a discount card you have from your favorite bakery, that gives you an amazing bargain and it would be a shame not to use it every morning while on your way to work, or the fact that you just went on a weekly shopping spree and you have to finish all the food and ready-meals you have bought before you can start eating better, you need to leave this kind of thinking behind and you simply have to understand your main goal and make no excuse this time. We all lie to ourselves, especially when it comes to being healthy and fit. We order another takeaway food because your favorite restaurant is offering a discount on a delivery app and you want to order just this one last time before making healthier decisions. You could start going to the gym, but it is really far from where you live, so you start coming up with excuses, to make yourself feel better. Maybe you have read about intermittent fasting before, but you also went and searched the bad stuff, the articles on intermittent fasting, that have no scientific or medical evidence behind them and it was probably a blog post made by someone, while drinking their morning coffee and having to come up with something to write about and then there is you, falling for it and thinking that you do not want to damage your health with such a serious and restricting diet. It is true that fasting is not made for everyone and it is true that living on a calorie deficit has still helped many people to achieve their goals, but many people do not understand or are not aware of the damage and the health risks behind that. With intermittent fasting, you will still be in a calorie deficit, if you do it right, but in a healthy calorie deficit. That is exactly why you should never consume less than 1200 calories while eating one meal a day because that right there is definitely starving and you can damage your health in a really bad way. Fasting is the safest, the healthiest, and the easiest way to do it, because it will become a norm for you and you will not go back to binge-eating and you will not want to go back to your previous eating habits ever again.

> *"Doctors won't make you healthy. Nutritionists won't make you slim. Teachers won't make you smart. Gurus won't make you calm. Mentors won't make you rich. Trainers won't make you fit. Ultimately, you have to take responsibility. Save yourself."*
>
> **– Naval Ravikant**

A 7-day plan

One thing is clear here, you have read this far, so you probably have thought about which route you want to take - which method would suit your lifestyle and eating habits the best, what to eat, and what not to eat. You have thrown all the ready-to-eat food out, you checked the condiments and how many sugars and bad carbs they contain, you have prepared your family for your new beginnings and you are ready to change your life and become the best version of yourself. But as we all know, any new beginnings are hard and we can get lost in all of it. Just to make things really understandable and you can kick-start your new life, you need to have a plan - two plans, to be exact. A daily plan and a meal plan. Remember, in order to achieve the best results, it is advisable to stick to clean eating and not indulge in too many cheat days and cheat meals, so here is a 7-day meal plan that will give you a better understanding of where and how to start.

Day 1 of 16:8

You might have many doubts, or maybe you have really high expectations. You might have no idea what you are getting yourself into, or you may be excited and ready to commit to this more than anything else. This is your first day and you might want to take some before pictures, weigh yourself, write down how you feel, to compare it later.

If you woke up at 9 AM and the first thing you used to do was rush to the kitchen after your morning routine, then from today, you have a new routine. Start your day with plain, black coffee - forget about sugar and milk. Taste the richness of the coffee beans, explore the internet and check where your coffee comes from, understand the story behind it and it will taste so much different. At this point, you may be hungry and your stomach is growling. Your brain is giving you signals to just go and eat, but this day will be different - not easy, but different. You can start preparing your meal at 11 PM but do not taste everything while making it, stay away from the temptation and trust your gut feeling. It is important to have a variety of different nutrients and your plate needs some color. For your first intermittent fasting meal, you will be cooking a chicken casserole.

You need 2 boneless chicken breasts, ½ finely chopped onion, 3 sweet potatoes that have been chopped into little cubes, minced garlic, a cup of Brussel sprouts, salt, pepper, cumin seeds, paprika, thyme leaves, dried cranberries, sliced almonds, wild rice, and chicken broth - preferably low-sodium chicken broth. Season the chicken with salt and pepper and preheat the oven to 350 degrees. Take the chicken, add 1 tablespoon of extra-virgin olive oil and add that in a skillet with the seasoned chicken. Cook the chicken until it is golden brown, take it out, and let it sit for 10 minutes. You should have your vegetables ready by now and the chicken should be cut into smaller pieces. Place the vegetables in a cooking dish, season it well, add a thyme leaf and chicken broth in the dish and cook until the vegetables have softened. While that is cooking in the oven, cook your rice separately. Take a baking pan, then stir the chicken, vegetables, cranberries, and rice together, add more chicken broth and top it with almonds. Cook for about 15 to 18 minutes and there you have it - it should only take you approximately an hour - you and your family are going to love it and it will leave you feeling warm and fuzzy inside. If you are used to snacking during the day or grabbing something to eat after a few hours of your meal, try to wait till 3 PM and have a light snack, like plain greek yogurt with blueberries and raspberries.

You can add chia seeds or flax seeds as well. You can start preparing for dinner around 6 PM, so you can be done with cooking around 7 PM and done with eating at 8 PM. As bad as it sounds, you will be okay and you can definitely go without your late-night snack and have the best sleep ever because your digestive system will be so thankful for not making it work all night long. For dinner, you are having shrimp zoodles. Not noodles, but zoodles. Zucchini noodles.

Get it? All jokes aside, zoodles are an amazing alternative for noodles, and the most important thing here, they look awesome and are worth a food post on your social media. You can use a vegetable peeler, a spiralizer, or shred the zucchini with a grater, to make them into thin-noodle-looking zoodles. For this, you will need some butter, about 3-4 tablespoons. As well as heavy cream, minced garlic, grated Parmesan cheese, freshly chopped parsley, 1 large, spiralized zucchini, fresh shrimp, salt, pepper and a cup of cherry tomatoes. Take 1 tablespoon of butter, melt it in the pan and add seasoned shrimp. Cook the shrimp until it turns pink, it will take you about 2 minutes for each side. When the shrimp is ready, take it out, but leave the shrimpy-buttery sauce in the pan. Take some more butter, add it to the pan and add your fresh, minced garlic, then whisk in heavy cream. Let that heat up, add cherry tomatoes, fresh parsley, grate some Parmesan in. Wait for about 3 minutes until the sauce has thickened, put the shrimp back in and add your zoodles, stir it all together and let the zoodles cook for about 1 minute, combine everything together and your shrimp zoodle dish is ready. Feel free to have a glass of wine, dark chocolate, and some roasted almonds, but make sure you are done by 8 PM.

On the second day, you are bound to wake up feeling energized. You probably woke up feeling like you have done a great job at fighting the late-night snack monster and you were able to get some good sleep. You could go for a nice breakfast, but you could also let your body deal with last night's feast and drink your water, coffee, or tea in peace. Water will become your best friend and as much as you want to add some fresh lemon to it, I would advise not to, but it will not break your fast, so this one is up to you. Let your body get rid of all the toxins, burn fat and improve your immune system just by doing absolutely nothing. Be patient until 11 PM, when you can start preparing your meal again. You might be missing your favorite breakfast meals and honestly, no one said you cannot have a breakfast meal at 12 PM, so today you are going to have a delicious late breakfast. You are going to have fluffy banana protein pancakes. You will need your favorite protein powder, 1 ripe and mashed banana, 2 eggs, baking powder, coconut oil, maple syrup, sliced banana, and strawberries. Get two bowls, separate the egg yolks from the whites and mix the eggs with a mixer until it forms into soft peaks. Add the mashed banana, ¼ tablespoon of baking powder, and 1 scoop of protein powder to the bowl with egg yolks and mix it all together until smooth consistency. Add half of the egg-white mixture to the egg-yolk mixture, gently stir it and then add the rest of the egg-white mixture and combine it. Get coconut oil, heat it in a skillet and start forming pancakes - pour the batter into the pan and bake until golden brown from both sides. You can top it with whip cream without sugar and add the berries on top instead, or maple syrup and the fresh berries. This meal will keep you satisfied until your next meal, but it is okay to have a snack in between, to avoid overeating for your dinner. You can have an oat bar, apple slices with peanut butter, or fresh guacamole with a handful of vegetable chips - carrot chips, beetroot chips, or eggplant chips. Remind yourself to drink water throughout the day, have a cup of green tea as well and it will help you with feeling less hungry, so you can wait for dinner and not feel like you are starving. For dinner, you are having one of the best options you could have - fish. Tonight, it will be salmon - rich in Omega-3 fatty acids, high in vitamin B, and is a great source of protein as well. You should consider making a salmon stir fry with green beans and mushrooms, but you will also need soy sauce, minced ginger and minced garlic, green onion, sesame oil, and of course, salmon fillet and quinoa. You want to have some fresh lemon as well, so you can squeeze lemon juice on top of the dish if you want.

Take your salmon fillet, cut it into cubes, put it in a bowl and add 2 tablespoons of soy sauce - you will marinate it while cutting other ingredients, let that sit aside. Cut the mushrooms and green beans into smaller pieces, prepare quinoa. Heat your skillet or a wok pan, add sesame oil, garlic, ginger, and the main ingredient - salmon and cook it for about 10 minutes until the salmon is fully cooked. When that is ready, put it aside and take your mushrooms and green beans, put them in the pan, you may take sesame seeds as well, if you have them, and roast them alongside the vegetables. Add the cooked quinoa, salmon and stir it all together. This meal is low in carbs and low in calories, but high in protein and calcium. Try not to have a snack after dinner every day, but if you feel like you might get a really bad craving later on and that will make you go look for something at night, try to have it before 8 PM. You can have nuts, cucumber slices with hummus, cherry tomatoes with mozzarella cheese, baby carrots, or roasted edamame beans, it is up to you. The bottom line is, do not go for something really heavy and high in fat after you just had your nutritious dinner.

Day 3 of 16:8

You have made it to day three and you should be really proud of yourself. You have not disappointed yourself and you stuck to your promises and you feel really good about these changes. You might want to get on the scales already, but wait some more, do not rush - let your body do its job, you just need to stick to your promises. I bet you are starting to enjoy the rich, delicious taste of black coffee and you have learned to drink tea too, even if tea was never really involved in your daily routine. You feel lighter, you feel better, you have been able to sleep through the whole night without waking up, you are less irritated and you generally find yourself feeling better. But since you have been doing so great, you might want to reward yourself and feel like you deserve some comfort food, something that might not be the best for you, but you have been sticking to fasting for 16 hours and you are on day three, so you know what, go for it.

Wait until 12 PM and have whatever your heart wishes. Whether it is a burger with fries and chicken nuggets on the side and a large coke, go for it. Do not restrict yourself, just stick to eating during your feeding window and you are more than good to go. Enjoy the freedom, enjoy the food, and do not think about anything else. As long as you drink lots of water during the day, you are doing great. If you want to cook something for dinner for the whole family, bake a large, cheesy pizza with crispy dough made from scratch. You will need 1 teaspoon of active dry yeast, ¼ teaspoon of white sugar, ¾ cup of lukewarm water, 2 cups of all-purpose flour, ½ teaspoon of salt. Take the yeast and dissolve it in hot water, add sugar to the mixture. It should take about 5 to 8 minutes for the yeast to form into a creamy foam texture. Mix 1 ¾ cup flour and salt into another bowl, pour in the yeast mixture and mix it until the dough seems ready enough. Have a floured surface ready and roll out your dough until it is smooth, keep kneading, and add more flour if it gets sticky. Roll it out in a circle or whatever shape you want and put it in a greased pan. Spread tomato sauce all over the pizza dough, take cherry tomatoes, basil leaves, mozzarella cheese, olives, and put it on top of the pizza. Bake until golden brown and the crust is crispy. If you want a pepperoni pizza, take slices of pepperoni, grated mozzarella cheese, fresh oregano, fresh onion rings, bell pepper, mushrooms and top it as you wish, you may grate some more cheese on top - the more cheese, the better, right? Enjoy your pizza night with a great movie, make sure to go to sleep early, get some great sleep. If you have trouble falling asleep, imagine yourself in a few months if you continue sticking to your goals and eventually get completely used to this fasting lifestyle, to the point where you feel like this is not even fasting anymore, it is your life now.

Day 4, or let's take it up a notch

Almost a full week. Not yet, but you are almost there. You did 16:8 for three days, I think it is only fair to make it a little bit harder for you. Not to make your life hard, but to let you try it out and see how you feel. You will have one meal today, you will be trying the famous OMAD (One Meal a Day) and no, you will not be taken to the hospital - actually, you will have so much energy, you will be able to run to your nearest hospital, run around the hospital 5 times, come back home and jump over your fence instead of opening it. Do not do that, but I am just warning you, you will have some serious energy today and you should take full advantage of it. If you eat around 12 PM, the usual time, it might be hard for you to get through the day, and starting from 5-6 PM you might feel pretty miserable. Full with energy, but really, really hungry. Since this is probably your first time trying to eat one meal a day, you should try to go until 4 PM at least and close your feeding window by 5 PM. Since you ate at 8 PM last night and then eat at 4 PM today, you have done 20 hours of fasting already. Make sure to drink loads of water until your eating window comes and keep yourself busy and occupied.

What to eat when you are having just one meal a day? You are going to have a variety of foods to get all the nutrients you need for the day and it will be at least 1200 calories or more. You should start easy since you are only eating at 4 PM, drink a cup of delicious bone broth, add some fresh herbs to it and wait for at least 10 minutes to have a proper meal. Prepare some potatoes, broccoli, and eggplant, cut everything into smaller pieces, season it with extra-virgin olive oil, add some coriander, dill, parsley, or any seasoning of your choice and mix it all together, then transfer it to a baking dish and put it in the oven until the vegetables are cooked.

Take ground turkey meat, chopped onion, minced garlic, bell pepper, and sweet corn, sautée all of it on the pan until the meat is thoroughly cooked. Once the roasted vegetables are ready, serve it on the plate, add the meat and the rest of the stuff on the side, dice some fresh cucumber and tomato and have a plate full of filling, delicious and nutritious food. You might want to use the last 5-10 minutes and have a dessert if you still have space for it, but do not force it if you feel really full. You can have a drink of your choice, whether it is lemon water, a latte, orange juice, a cold, sparkly drink - this is up to you. You will feel full, but you should not consume less than 1000 calories. Ideally, you should have about 1200-1500 calories, and sometimes it might be difficult to even consume that much, but if you are missing calories, you can have a bulletproof coffee (coffee with butter) that is about 300 calories per cup, or a mocha frappé that can contain even 700 calories alone, so this is where some calorie counting might come in handy.

As soon as the clock hits 5 PM, you should focus on having water, tea, or plain coffee only, no more calories for the night, you are letting your body restart fully. Make sure you write down how you feel, take notes, ask your family members if they have noticed any mood changes or unusual behavior.

Day 5

Having one meal a day was pretty tough, so no more of that for now. You have to be patient until 4 PM and then you can have a 4-hour eating window and stop eating at your usual 8 PM, so you can get back into the 16:8 method easily. Make those 4 hours count and have two lighter meals and a snack - today it will be an avocado salad at 4 PM, a snack at 6 PM, and quesadillas for dinner at 7 PM. For the avocado salad, you will need ripe avocado, cucumber, cherry tomatoes, honey, garlic, red onion, fresh parsley, cilantro, and lemon. Start with the salad dressing and whisk lemon juice, cilantro, parsley, and honey into a bowl. Cut the onions, avocado, tomatoes, and cucumbers, add them to the same bowl and mix it all together, add salt and pepper to taste. Very easy, very nutritious, and light, very quick to make. For your snack, cut a ripe mango into small cubes and cut up 1 banana, this will keep you going until dinner time, while you are preparing your quesadillas. For these, you will need boneless, skinless chicken breast, shredded cheddar cheese, sour cream, green onions, bell peppers, flour tortillas, shredded Monterey jack cheese, one sliced avocado, vegetable oil, extra-virgin olive oil, salt, pepper, chili powder, and dried oregano. Cut your green onions, bell peppers, make sure you have your spices ready and you can start with heating up the pan and adding olive oil. Start by adding bell peppers, onions, season it with salt and pepper, and cook until soft. Take it out of the pan and put it aside, it is time to cook the chicken. Season it with chili powder, salt, and pepper, and cook until golden brown and fully cooked from both sides. Put the chicken away and take 1 tortilla, place it on the pan, sprinkle both of the cheeses on top, add the cooked chicken, a few slices of avocado, and the green onion. Fold the tortilla over and cook until the bottom gets brown, flip it, and cook the other half. Slice the quesadilla into wedges, add some sour cream on top and that is it, dinner is served. Make sure you are finished by 8 PM and go back to your regular routine. Stay hydrated, stay patient and focus on the goal.

The weekend

If you started on a Monday, like all of us do when it comes to dieting and being healthy, it is a Saturday and you are probably enjoying the weekend at home with your family and that means food, food, and more food. If you want to enjoy a nice breakfast with the family, have eggs, bacon, grits, hash browns, waffles, and pancakes for breakfast at 10 AM, it is fine. If you start eating before your eating window, you can have dinner at 5 PM, finish eating at 6 PM and just wait until the next day, when you can enjoy a beautiful Sunday breakfast in the garden, or on your balcony and eat whatever you want, while feeling completely guilt-free, because intermittent fasting is not about restricting yourself, it is an extremely flexible way of life, just in a healthier way. Do not miss out on some family time, cook in the morning and eat whatever you wish, because you will still be losing weight and benefitting from fasting.

As you can see, there are more pros than cons here. It will not be easy to stay away from food sometimes, but you can make it work and you can fulfill your goals by making small adjustments. Intermittent fasting does not have to be difficult, it is all about planning your time and being mindful.

Conclusion

With all of this in mind, it is time to start applying everything you have read and learned about intermittent fasting. Most likely, you have thought about real-life situations - your life situations, where involving fasting could be difficult, but you have started to plan it out. This book has given you new ideas, new motivation, possibly a new way of thinking and it is your job to take what you can, adjust it if needed, and apply it. The person you are now while reading this book, will not be the same person if you start practicing intermittent fasting at this instant. Besides the obvious weight loss, health improvement, beautiful, glowing and healthy skin, and a new wardrobe, you will also train your mind and develop a new mindset. You will be able to give advice to your friends, colleagues, or family members and take your experience as a great example and help them in their journey. Understanding your bad eating habits - that a change is needed - and that you do not want to end up with serious health condition sounds beautiful, but it is hard to do in real life. If you can do it now and achieve your goals, even if you doubt yourself, you will become an inspiration for others. Some people have made intermittent fasting their life and after going through it all on their own, the ups and the downs, the hardships, understanding what works and what does not, they have made a career out of it. They have made it their whole life, they are teaching and helping others that have no idea where to start.

Some people have no idea they can do it, you can be the person to change that, just like this book can change you. Forget about the quick fixes and the diets that will never help and focus on something that is sustainable, like intermittent fasting is. You will lose weight quickly, but the real change will start to be noticeable in a few months, from the portion size you can eat, to your skin never breaking out again, to fast metabolism that will help you to maintain your weight, to the low blood sugar levels, a healthy heart and no serious health condition risks. If you think about it, losing weight is probably the easiest thing to do here, as it will come on its own, while you are probably here thinking it will be the hardest. It will be hard to stay away from food when you need to, but it will not be hard to lose weight once you do it. And once you see the weight coming off, psychologically, you will not break your fast sooner than you should, because you will love the results and what comes with dedication and staying on the right track. Everyone that does intermittent fasting always talks about it as a lifestyle, not a diet. They come for weight loss and stay for the health benefits.

This book was written with pure intentions, from personal experiences, and is meant for you to understand that this journey does not have to be hard, at least not as hard as you think it would be. It will be an interesting transition for you and you will notice how you evolve and change.

Most importantly, you will recognize the hard work and dedication you have put into this when you have finally reached your goal.

"The job of fasting is to supply the body with the ideal environment to accomplish its work of healing."

- Joel Fuhrman

References

American Heart Association. 2019. Regular fasting could lead to a longer, healthier life.

https://www.heart.org/en/news/2019/11/25/regular-fasting-could-lead-to-longer-healthier-life

Sutton, EF., Bey, R., Early, KS. et.al., 2018. Cell Metabolism.

https://www.sciencedirect.com/science/article/pii/S1550413118302535

Trepanowski, JF., Kroeger, CM., Barnosky, A. et al. 2017. Effect of Alternate-Day Fasting on Weight Loss, Weight Maintenance, and Cardioprotection Among Metabolically Healthy Obese Adults: A Randomized Clinical Trial. JAMA Intern Med. 2017;177(7):930–938.

doi:10.1001/jamainternmed.2017.0936

World Health Organisation. 2020. Obesity and Overweight. https://www.who.int/news-room/fact-sheets/detail/obesity-and-overweight

Gîlcă, M., Soian, I., Mohora, M., Petec, C., Muscurel, C., Dinu, V. 2003. The effect of fasting on the parameters of the antioxidant defense system in the blood of vegetarian human subjects.

Rom J Intern Med. 2003;41(3):283-92. PMID: 15526512.

Vieira, A., Costa, R., Macedo, R., Coconcelli, L., & Kruel, L. 2016. Effects of aerobic exercise performed in the fasted v. fed state on fat and carbohydrate metabolism in adults: A systematic review and meta-analysis. British Journal of Nutrition, 116(7), 1153-1164. doi:10.1017/S0007114516003160

Dansinger, M. 2019. Type 1 Diabetes. https://www.webmd.com/diabetes/type-1-diabetes

Albosta, M., Bakke, J. 2021. Intermittent fasting: is there a role in the treatment of diabetes? A review of the literature and guide for primary care physicians. Clin

Diabetes Endocrinol 7, 3. https://doi.org/10.1186/s40842-020-00116-1

Griffith, T., Chun, C. 2018. Fasting and Cancer. https://www.healthline.com/health/fasting-and-cancer

Mattson, M. 2005. Energy Intake, Meal Frequency, and Health: A Neurobiological Perspective.

Annual Review of Nutrition 2005 25:1, 237-260. https://www.annualreviews.org/action/showCitFormats?doi=10.1146%2Fannurev.nutr.25.050304

.092526

Vieira, A., Costa, R., Macedo, R., Coconcelli, L., & Kruel, L. 2016. Effects of aerobic exercise performed in the fasted v. fed state on fat and carbohydrate metabolism in adults: A systematic review and meta-analysis. British Journal of Nutrition, 116(7), 1153-1164. doi:10.1017/S0007114516003160

Ezzat Faris, M., Hussein, R., Ahmad Al-Kurd, A., et.al. 2012. Impact of Ramadan Intermittent Fasting on Oxidative Stress Measured by Urinary 15--Isoprostane, Journal of Nutrition and Metabolism, vol. 2012, Article

ID 802924, 9 pages. https://doi.org/10.1155/2012/802924

Di Biase, S., Lee, C., Brandhorst, S., et.al. 2016. Fasting-Mimicking Diet Reduces HO-1 to Promote T Cell-Mediated Tumor Cytotoxicity. Longo publishers. https://doi.org/10.1016/j.ccell.2016.06.005

Tith, R., Bilodeau-Bertrand, M., Lee, G., et.al. 2019. Fasting during Ramadan Increases Risk of Very Preterm Birth among Arabic-Speaking Women, The Journal of Nutrition, Volume 149, Issue 10, Pages 1826–1832.

https://doi.org/10.1093/jn/nxz126